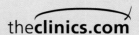

MAGNETIC RESONANCE IMAGING CLINICS

Breast MR Imaging

Guest Editor

CHRISTIANE K. KUHL, MD

August 2006 • Volume 14 • Number 3

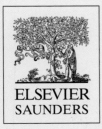

ELSEVIER SAUNDERS

An imprint of Elsevier, Inc
PHILADELPHIA LONDON TORONTO MONTREAL SYDNEY TOKYO

W.B. SAUNDERS COMPANY
A Divison of Elsevier Inc.

Elsevier Inc. ● 1600 John F. Kennedy Boulevard ● Suite 1800 ●
Philadelphia, Pennsylvania 19103-2899

http://www.mri.theclinics.com

MRI CLINICS OF NORTH AMERICA Volume 14, Number 3
August 2006 ISSN 1064-9689, ISBN 1-4160-3531-1

Editor: Barton Dudlick

Reprints: For copies of 100 or more, of articles in this publication, please contact the Commercial
Reprints Department, Elsevier Inc., 360 Park Avenue South, New York, New York 10010-1710. Tel.
(212) 633-3813, Fax: (212) 462-1935, email: reprints@elsevier.com.

The ideas and opinions expressed in *Magnetic Resonance Imaging Clinics of North America* do not
necessarily reflect those of the Publisher. The Publisher does not assume any responsibility for
any injury and/or damage to persons or property arising out of or related to any use of the
material contained in this periodical. The reader is advised to check the appropriate medical
literature and the product information currently provided by the manufacturer of each drug to be
administered to verify the dosage, the method and duration of administration, or
contraindications. It is the responsibility of the treating physician or other health care
professional, relying on independent experience and knowledge of the patient, to determine drug
dosages and the best treatment for the patient. Mention of any product in this issue should not be
construed as endorsement by the contributors, editors, or the Publisher of the product or
manufacturers' claims.

Magnetic Resonance Imaging Clinics of North America (ISSN 1064-9689) is published quarterly by
Elsevier Inc., 360 Park Avenue South, New York, NY 10010-1710. Months of issue are February,
May, August, and November. Business and Editorial Offices: 1600 John F. Kennedy Blvd., Suite
1800, Philadelphia, PA 19103-2899. Customer Service Office: 6277 Sea Harbor Drive, Orlando,
FL 32887-4800. Periodicals postage paid at New York, NY and additional mailing offices.
Subscription prices are $226.00 per year (US individuals), $336.00 per year (US institutions),
$110.00 per year (US students), $253.00 per year (Canadian individuals), $413.00 per year
(Canadian institutions), $149.00 per year (Canadian students), $308.00 per year (international
individuals), $413.00 per year (international institutions), and $149.00 per year (international
students). International air speed delivery is included in all *Clinics* subscription prices. All prices
are subject to change without notice. **POSTMASTER:** Send address changes to *Magnetic
Resonance Imaging Clinics*, Elsevier Periodicals Customer Service, 6277 Sea Harbor Drive,
Orlando, FL 32887-4800. **Customer Service: 1-800-654-2452 (US). From outside of the US,
call 1-407-345-4000.**

Magnetic Resonance Imaging Clinics of North America is covered in the *RSNA Index of Imaging
Literature, Index Medicus, MEDLINE,* and *EMBASE/Excerpta Medica.*

Printed in the United States of America.

BREAST MR IMAGING

GUEST EDITOR

CHRISTIANE K. KUHL, MD
Professor of Radiology, Department of Radiology,
University of Bonn, Bonn, Germany

CONTRIBUTORS

FRIEDEMANN BAUM, MD
Women's Health Care Center, Diagnostisches
Brustzentrum Göttingen, Germany

UWE FISCHER, MD
Professor, Women's Health Care Center,
Diagnostisches Brustzentrum Göttingen, Germany

DANIEL FLOERY, MD
Department of Radiology, Medical University
of Vienna, Vienna, Austria

GARY FREEDMAN, MD
Member, Radiation Oncology; and Associate
Director, Breast Evaluation Center, Fox Chase
Cancer Center, Philadelphia, Pennsylvania

THOMAS H. HELBICH, MD
Department of Radiology, Medical University
of Vienna, Vienna, Austria

BRUCE J. HILLMAN, MD
Theodore E. Keats Professor of Radiology,
Department of Radiology; and Department
of Public Health Sciences, University of Virginia,
Charlottesville, Virginia; Network Chair, American
College of Radiology Imaging Network,
Philadelphia, Pennsylvania

NOLA HYLTON, PhD
Professor of Radiology, Department of Radiology,
and Director, Magnetic Resonance Science Center,
University of California, San Francisco, California

CHRISTIANE K. KUHL, MD
Professor of Radiology, Department of Radiology,
University of Bonn, Bonn, Germany

LAURA LIBERMAN MD, FACR
Director of Breast Imaging Section, Department
of Radiology, Memorial Sloan-Kettering Cancer
Center; Attending Radiologist, Memorial Hospital;
Professor of Radiology, Department of Radiology,
Weill Medical College of Cornell University, New
York, New York

SUSANNE LUFTNER-NAGEL, MD
Women's Health Care Center, Diagnostisches
Brustzentrum Göttingen, Germany

ELIZABETH A. MORRIS, MD
Associate Professor of Radiology, Weill Medical
College of Cornell University; and Associate
Radiologist, Department of Radiology, Memorial
Sloan-Kettering Cancer Center, New York,
New York

MONICA MORROW, MD
G. Willing Pepper Chair in Cancer Research;
and Chairman, Department of Surgical Oncology;
and Senior Member, Fox Chase Cancer Center;
Professor of Surgery, Temple University,
Philadelphia, Pennsylvania

SUSAN OREL, MD
Department of Radiology, Hospital of the
University of Pennsylvania, Philadelphia,
Pennsylvania

MITCHELL SCHNALL, MD, PhD
Department of Radiology, Hospital of the
University of Pennsylvania, Philadelphia,
Pennsylvania

BREAST MR IMAGING

Volume 14 · Number 3 · August 2006

Contents

The American College of Radiology Breast Imaging and Reporting Data System MR imaging lexicon incorporates morphologic and kinetic features of lesions identified on breast MR imaging. This brief article is aimed at introducing this material and should not be used as a definitive guide. Because the breast MR imaging lexicon is a work in progress, there are many areas that need exploring and better characterization. It is hoped that the radiologist uses the terms and concepts presented here as a template to which future lexicon terminology can be added.

There is broad agreement in that breast MR imaging, compared with all other contemporary breast imaging techniques, offers the highest sensitivity for primary and recurrent invasive breast cancer. For a long time, however, the modality suffered from the reputation of offering only a limited specificity. In addition, the allegedly low sensitivity for intraductal breast cancer hampered the more widespread use of breast MR imaging. More recent results, however, suggest that the specificity and positive predictive value of breast MR imaging are at least equivalent to those of mammography and that the sensitivity for ductal carcinoma in situ (DCIS) is at least comparable to mammography, if not higher. Apart from increasing reader experience, this progress is mainly attributable to the fact that in parallel with improved MR imaging technology, more refined interpretation criteria became available. These criteria allow a substantially improved diagnosis of malignant masses and of DCIS. This article provides an overview on the current status of the diagnostic criteria that are used for differential diagnosis in breast MR imaging and on the diagnostic accuracy that is achievable with breast MR imaging.

Breast MR Imaging in the Diagnostic Setting

Mitchell Schnall and Susan Orel

The role of MR imaging as an adjunct in the diagnostic evaluation of findings on mammography or clinical examination continues to evolve. Clearly, the use of MR imaging to evaluate all suspicious screening findings is not reasonable or effective. In particular, the role of MR imaging in the setting of mammographic microcalcifications is limited. MR imaging may be used in cases of one or more mammographically detected masses or asymmetric density in an effort to avoid biopsy. Optimized MR imaging technique; careful mammography, ultrasound, and MR imaging correlation; and adherence to interpretation guidelines are important to avoid false-negative diagnoses.

Breast MR Imaging in Assessing Extent of Disease

Laura Liberman

Breast MR imaging is valuable in assessment of extent of disease in the ipsilateral and contralateral breast in women who have breast cancer. In the ipsilateral breast, MR imaging depicts otherwise unsuspected sites of cancer in 16% (range, 6%–34%). In the contralateral breast, MR imaging depicts otherwise unsuspected sites of cancer in 6% (range, 3%–24%). MR imaging is most likely to depict additional sites of cancer in women with invasive lobular cancer and a family history of breast cancer. MR imaging can also assist in evaluating involvement of skin, pectoral muscle, and chest wall. Disadvantages of breast MR imaging include cost and additional procedures (follow-up and biopsy); furthermore, no data as yet show that breast MR imaging in the extent of disease evaluation improves disease-free or overall survival. If breast MR imaging is used in evaluating extent of disease, it is necessary to have the capability to perform biopsy of lesions detected by MR imaging only.

Preoperative MR Imaging in Patients with Breast Cancer: Preoperative Staging, Effects on Recurrence Rates, and Outcome Analysis

Uwe Fischer, Friedemann Baum, and Susanne Luftner-Nagel

As well documented for other diseases (ie, lymphoma), an accurate pretherapeutic assessment of the extent of breast cancer is essential for planning the appropriate treatment to get the best long-term results, decrease recurrence rates, and increase patient survival. This article presents an overview of the effects of preoperative local staging with MR imaging in breast cancer patients.

A Clinical Oncology Perspective on the Use of Breast MR

Monica Morrow and Gary Freedman

MR imaging of the breast detects additional carcinoma in as many as 30% of women thought to have localized disease by clinical examination and mammography. This has led some to advocate its routine use in the preoperative evaluation of breast cancer patients. However, local failure rates in patients selected for breast conservation by conventional methods are less than 5% at 10 years, suggesting that the majority of this disease is controlled with radiotherapy. The potential role of MR in the preoperative evaluation and postoperative follow-up of patients with early-stage breast cancer is discussed.

The traditional methods for selecting women for breast conservation therapy (BCT), coupled with adjuvant radiation therapy, have reduced recurrence rates of BCT to acceptable levels. These recurrence rates are still significant, however. They may be further affected by the application of more anatomically targeted radiation therapy. Preoperative MR imaging should theoretically reduce the local failure rate of BCT by at least 5%, with only a modest increase in the mastectomy rate. The evolution of BCT to include more targeted radiation therapy and ablation should place an even larger emphasis on accurate tumor localization and has the potential to allow BCT to become more prevalent and effective.

Contrast-enhanced MR imaging is being used increasingly because of its high sensitivity to breast cancer and superior ability to demonstrate the extent and distribution of disease. In addition to this direct clinical use, MR imaging in the neoadjuvant treatment setting allows exploration of its potential value in quantifying primary tumor response. The high sensitivity and staging accuracy of MR imaging may yield more accurate classification of objective tumor response using RECIST criteria than clinical examination or mammography. Functional measurements hold the promise of greater sensitivity for detecting biologic effects of targeted treatments than simple anatomic methods.

The adequate management of individuals who carry a high lifetime risk for breast cancer is still an unsettled issue. This holds especially true for subjects with documented or suspected germline mutation of a breast cancer susceptibility gene. These women face a lifetime risk for breast cancer of up to 80%, which is, of course, significant. Still, this means that approximately one fifth of women never develop the disease. The perceived mutilating effects of preventive mastectomy make the decision for surgical prevention difficult for most women. Secondary prevention aims at identifying familial breast cancer at the earliest possible stage. During recent years, considerable evidence has been accumulated that breast MR imaging is substantially more sensitive than mammography and breast ultrasound regarding the identification of familial breast cancer. It should be considered an integral part of a surveillance program for women at increased familial risk for breast cancer, be it with or without documented mutation of a breast cancer susceptibility gene.

MR imaging of the breast has been shown to identify breast cancers that have gone undetected by mammography. There are a number of potential designs that can be used to further evaluate breast MR imaging, particularly with respect to its impact on clinical care. Determination of whether using breast MR imaging to screen healthy individuals for breast cancer actually reduces breast cancer–specific mortality—and whether this can be accomplished at an acceptable cost—probably requires randomized, controlled clinical.

MR imaging of the breast allows the detection of suspicious breast lesions that are occult at mammography and ultrasound. For the histologic verification of such lesions, percutaneous MR imaging–guided biopsy techniques can now be offered as an alternative to open breast biopsy. This review focuses on the currently available devices and techniques for MR imaging–guided percutaneous breast biopsy and reports their achievable diagnostic accuracy. Technical success rates and strategies for patient management are also outlined. In addition, new developments in MR imaging–guided minimally invasive therapeutic interventions are discussed, as well as the potential for research opportunities and directions.

FORTHCOMING ISSUES

RECENT ISSUES

THE CLINICS ARE NOW AVAILABLE ONLINE!

Access your subscription at:
www.theclinics.com

GOAL STATEMENT

The goal of *Magnetic Resonance Imaging Clinics of North America* is to keep practicing radiologists and radiology residents up to date with current clinical practice in radiology by providing timely articles reviewing the state of the art in patient care.

ACCREDITATION

The *Magnetic Resonance Imaging Clinics of North America* is planned and implemented in accordance with the Essential Areas and Policies of the Accreditation Council for Continuing Medical Education (ACCME) through the joint sponsorship of the University of Virginia School of Medicine and Elsevier. The University of Virginia School of Medicine is accredited by the ACCME to provide continuing medical education for physicians.

The University of Virginia School of Medicine designates this educational activity for a maximum of 60 *AMA PRA Category 1 Credits™*. Physicians should only claim credit commensurate with the extent of their participation in the activity.

The American Medical Association has determined that physicians not licensed in the US who participate in this CME activity are eligible for *AMA PRA Category 1 Credits™*.

Credit can be earned by reading the text material, taking the CME examination online at http://www.theclinics.com/home/cme, and completing the evaluation. After taking the test, you will be required to review any and all incorrect answers. Following completion of the test and evaluation, your credit will be awarded and you may print your certificate.

FACULTY DISCLOSURE/CONFLICT OF INTEREST

The University of Virginia School of Medicine, as an ACCME accredited provider, endorses and strives to comply with the Accreditation Council for Continuing Medical Education (ACCME) Standards of Commercial Support, Commonwealth of Virginia statutes, University of Virginia policies and procedures, and associated federal and private regulations and guidelines on the need for disclosure and monitoring of proprietary and financial interests that may affect the scientific integrity and balance of content delivered in continuing medical education activities under our auspices.

The University of Virginia School of Medicine requires that all CME activities accredited through this institution be developed independently and be scientifically rigorous, balanced and objective in the presentation/discussion of its content, theories and practices.

All authors/editors participating in an accredited CME activity are expected to disclose to the readers relevant financial relationships with commercial entities occurring within the past 12 months (such as grants or research support, employee, consultant, stock holder, member of speakers bureau, etc.). The University of Virginia School of Medicine will employ appropriate mechanisms to resolve potential conflicts of interest to maintain the standards of fair and balanced education to the reader. Questions about specific strategies can be directed to the Office of Continuing Medical Education, University of Virginia School of Medicine, Charlottesville, Virginia.

The authors/editors listed below have identified no financial or professional relationships for themselves or their spouse/partner:
Friedemann Baum, MD; Barton Dudlick (Acquistions Editor); Uwe Fischer, MD; Daniel Floery, MD; Gary Freedman, MD; Bruce J. Hillman, MD; Nola Hylton, PhD; Christiane K. Kuhl, MD (Guest Editor); Laura Liberman, MD, FACR; Susanne Luftner-Nagel, MD; Elizabeth A. Morris, MD; Monica Morrow, MD; and Susan Orel, MD.

The authors/editors listed below have identified the following professional or financial affiliations for themselves or their spouse/partner:

Thomas H. Helbich, MD is an independent contractor for GE and Ethicon.
Mitchell Schnall, MD, PhD is on the speaker's bureau for Siemen's Medical; is on the speaker's bureau and the advisory board for Berley.

Disclosure of Discussion of Non-FDA Approved Uses for Pharmaceutical and/or Medical Devices.
The University of Virginia School of Medicine, as an ACCME provider, requires that all authors identify and disclose any "off label" uses for pharmaceutical and medical device products. The University of Virginia School of Medicine recommends that each physician fully review all the available data on new products or procedures prior to clinical use.

TO ENROLL

To enroll in the Magnetic Resonance Imaging Clinics of North America Continuing Medical Education program, call customer service at 1-800-654-2452 or visit us online at www.theclinics.com/home/cme. The CME program is available to subscribers for an additional fee of $175.00

ELSEVIER
SAUNDERS

MAGNETIC
RESONANCE
IMAGING CLINICS

Magn Reson Imaging Clin N Am 14 (2006) xi–xii

Preface

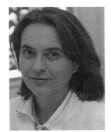

Christiane K. Kuhl, MD
Guest Editor

Christiane K. Kuhl, MD
Professor of Radiology
Department of Radiology
University of Bonn
Sigmund-Freud-Strasse 25, D-53105
Bonn, Germany

E-mail address:
kuhl@uni-bonn.de

For a long time, breast MR imaging was considered a second- or third-line imaging modality with questionable benefit for the patient. It was considered a high-priced way to approach diagnostic problems that could have easier been settled by core biopsy as well, and as a diagnostic test that would often cause more problems than it would solve. The multitude of imaging protocols was hardly comprehensible even for the MR expert and led to a similarly huge variety of diagnostic criteria for interpreting breast MR imaging studies. It was generally agreed on that this technique was sensitive—but how should the extra sensitivity be exploited to the advantage of the patient in view of the absence of techniques for MR-guided tissue sampling?

Fortunately, over the last decade, the field has made substantial progress. Although breast MR imaging is still a cost-intensive modality, it has made its way into clinical practice. The breast is the one MR application with the steepest growth rates. This change has occurred due to several major advances. The most important breakthrough was the publication of the MR BI-RADS lexicon (see the article by Morris) that, in turn, paved the way to a more standardized universally acceptable approach to breast MR image acquisition and image interpretation (see the article by Kuhl). Another major step was the development of techniques for MR-guided biopsy, in particular MR-guided vacuum-assisted core biopsy (see the article by Floery and Helbich). Lastly, the role of breast MR imaging has changed over the past years. Its use is no longer restricted to the "rule out recurrent cancer" situation or to clarify an equivocal mammographic finding. It has now been expanded to include patients with a normal or benign mammogram but with an increased risk for breast cancer. This pertains to women with a strong family history of breast cancer, with or without documented mutation in a breast cancer susceptibility gene (see the article by Kuhl), or women who have received a tissue diagnosis that puts them at increased risk (such as lobular cancer in situ, radial scar). In addition, this group includes women with a recent diagnosis of breast cancer who undergo breast MR imaging for staging of the ipsilateral breast and screening of the opposite breast (see the articles by Liberman and Fischer and colleagues). In addition, more "functional" breast imaging techniques have been developed that

1064-9689/06/$ – see front matter © 2006 Elsevier Inc. All rights reserved.
mri.theclinics.com

doi:10.1016/j.mric.2006.10.001

improve the assessment of response to neoadjuvant chemotherapy (see the article by Hylton).

Whereas the use of breast MR imaging for screening women at familial risk for breast cancer has rapidly been adopted in clinical practice, its use for staging known breast cancer is still discussed controversially. Opponents argue that preoperative breast MR imaging will lead to a substantial increase of mastectomy rates owing to the additional conventionally occult multicentric breast cancers that will be diagnosed with MR imaging in as many as 26% of patients. The concern is that this may annihilate the advances that have been made over past decades regarding breast-conserving treatment. Because even without preoperative breast MR imaging, recurrence rates after breast conservation have been low, one may conclude that the additional lesions identified by MR imaging may be biologically irrelevant or sufficiently treated by postoperative radiotherapy. This perspective is presented in the article by Morrow.

Although this is a valid concern, some solid facts substantiate the recommendation to use breast MR imaging for staging patients with a biopsy-proven cancer who are amenable to breast-conserving treatment. These facts are outlined in the article by Schnall. Not withstanding the progress that has been made regarding adjuvant chemotherapy, and antihormonal or antibody treatment, surgery is still the mainstay of breast cancer therapy for local control and to avoid distant metastases. If it is agreeable that surgery is necessary, it is clear that one should use the most sensitive imaging modality that is available to map disease extent, which is clearly breast MR imaging. Mapping disease extent by MR imaging, CT, or even PET is common clinical practice and is considered an essential part of the pre-surgical treatment planning of virtually all other types of operable cancers, such as lung, liver, pancreas, bone, brain, and colorectal cancer. For the breast, radiotherapy may deal with small disseminated tumor cells, yet the additional cancers that are diagnosed by MR imaging alone have a considerable size. Indeed, these additional cancers seem to have the same size, histology, and biologic profile as the ones that have been diagnosed by mammography; therefore, there is no reason to assume that "MR only" disease is biologically irrelevant. This is also supported by long-term recurrence rates that have been shown to match closely with the rates of multicentric disease as detected by MR imaging at the primary diagnosis of breast cancer.

Still, the opponents may be right in that breast MR imaging may indeed cause an unnecessary increase of mastectomy rates; however, this increase is not an unavoidable consequence of breast MR imaging, per se. In fact, this increase happens if one makes the mistake of sticking to old paradigms and copying them to a new situation. The recommendation to perform mastectomy for multicentric disease stems from a time when mammography alone was used for local staging. This recommendation may not be adequate for the more subtle multicentric disease revealed by MR imaging. MR-diagnosed multicentric disease should probably not be treated according to the same practice guidelines that have been established for mammographically diagnosed multicentric cancer. Surgical guidelines will probably have to be modified to account for the higher sensitivity of MR imaging. It will take years before the results of prospective clinical trials are available if ever they will be done (see the article by Hillman). For the time being, we recommend that radiologists use their own sense of proportion when discussing treatment strategies for MR-diagnosed multicentric disease. Additional lumpectomies for the extra cancers detected by MR imaging may be a safe and tissue-sparing alternative to mastectomy. In some patients with very small additional lesions, one may even decide to follow the lesions ("watchful waiting") and see whether radiation and adjuvant therapy deal with them, especially if vacuum-assisted core biopsy has been used to establish the diagnosis. Although this approach may sound as if we put the patient at risk, any of these strategies will be less risky than the head-in-the-sand policy that is advocated implicitly if no staging breast MR imaging is offered in the first place.

Breast MR imaging is nothing but a tool. Having accurate information about the tumor burden in patients with operable breast cancer is important and, per se, cannot be "bad." Instead, the diligent and careful use of this information will determine whether, eventually, we do the patient good or harm.

ELSEVIER
SAUNDERS

MAGNETIC
RESONANCE
IMAGING CLINICS

Magn Reson Imaging Clin N Am 14 (2006) 293–303

Breast MR Imaging Lexicon Updated

Elizabeth A. Morris, MD[a,b,*]

- Need for standardization
- Characterization of benign and malignant
- Breast MR imaging technique
- Breast histopathology and MR imaging
- Background enhancement
- Description of morphologic features
  Focus
  Mass
  Shape and margins
- *Internal enhancement*
- *Nonmass enhancement*
- Description of kinetic features
- Predictive morphologic features
  Benign disease
  Malignant disease
- Suggested algorithm for interpretation
- Summary
- References

Breast MR imaging is an established technique for supplementing mammography and breast ultrasound in the imaging of breast disease. The power of breast MR imaging resides in the extreme sensitivity in the diagnosis of invasive breast malignancy. As is true with other breast imaging techniques, the specificity is not as high as the sensitivity, because enhancement alone is not sufficient for the determination of malignancy. Because breast MR imaging uses intravenous contrast, any area of increased vascularity is evident on the postcontrast images. The morphologic and enhancement parameters, including the kinetic uptake of the intravenous contrast material by the lesion, are essential to characterize an MR imaging–depicted lesion. By analyzing the morphology and kinetic behavior of a lesion, the specificity of breast MR imaging is improved. In this article, the morphologic and kinetic parameters of benign and malignant breast lesions are discussed. The American College of Radiology (ACR) Breast Imaging and Reporting Data System (BI-RADS) MR imaging lexicon describing architectural features and dynamic kinetic parameters is presented.

Need for standardization

During the past decade, as breast MR imaging has become incorporated into the clinical evaluation of the breast, it has become apparent that standardization of terminology is important. As with mammography, there should be concise, clear, and easily understood language used when describing a lesion seen on breast MR imaging so that the MR description can be understood without the benefit of looking at the actual image. The need for a standardized lexicon for analysis of findings identified on breast MR imaging is twofold: to describe the findings concisely so as to facilitate communication between radiologists and referring physicians and to allow analysis of outcomes across institutions so as to validate management recommendations.

A lexicon developed by an international working group of breast MR imaging experts was supported

[a] Weill Medical College of Cornell University, 1275 York Avenue, New York, NY 10021, USA
[b] Department of Radiology, Memorial Sloan-Kettering Cancer Center, 1275 York Avenue, New York, NY 10021, USA
* Department of Radiology, Memorial Sloan-Kettering Cancer Center, 1275 York Avenue, New York, NY 10021.
E-mail address: morrise@mskcc.org

1064-9689/06/$ – see front matter © 2006 Elsevier Inc. All rights reserved.   doi:10.1016/j.mric.2006.07.001
mri.theclinics.com

by the ACR to develop a consensus lexicon that would describe the findings that are seen on breast MR imaging [1–3]. The goal of the group was to arrive at a consensus regarding architectural and kinetic features that are seen on contrast-enhanced breast MR imaging. The lexicon was published in 2004. Terms that are used are listed in Box 1. The working group expressly tried to incorporate familiar language used in other BI-RADS lexicons [4]. When a BI-RADS descriptor could be used, it was applied to the corresponding finding on MR imaging. If a new descriptor was required, the descriptor was developed for findings unique to MR imaging. By virtue that breast MR imaging uses contrast and mammography does not, terms to describe the kinetic uptake of contrast by the lesion are unique to breast MR imaging. Similarly, aspects of morphologic analysis, such as pattern of enhancement, are unique to the breast MR imaging examination. The shape and margin analysis, however, is similar to the BI-RADS analysis used in mammography.

Box 1: Focus and/or foci

Mass: margin
Smooth
Irregular
Spiculated

Mass: shape
Oval
Round
Lobular
Irregular

Mass: enhancement
Homogeneous
Heterogeneous
Rim
Dark internal septation
Enhancing internal septations
Central enhancement

Nonmass enhancement
Focal area
Linear
Ductal
Segmental
Regional
Multiple regions
Diffuse

Nonmass enhancement internal enhancement
Homogeneous
Heterogeneous
Stippled/punctate
Clumped
Reticular/dendritic

Symmetric versus asymmetric for bilateral studies

Data from Refs. [1–3].

Characterization of benign and malignant

Lesion interpretation in breast MR imaging relies entirely on lesion enhancement. When analyzing a breast MR examination, the first step is to establish that the patient received an adequate dose of intravenous contrast. Although there are several sophisticated methods that can assess the presence of contrast, the simplest form of confirmation that contrast was received is that vessels in the breast are identified as enhancing structures.

Solely identifying an enhancing area on breast MR imaging as suspicious does not optimize the specificity of breast MR imaging and results in too many false-positive biopsies. For the best analysis, all features of the lesion should be analyzed, including kinetics as well as morphology of enhancement. By combining kinetic and morphologic information with clinical history and conventional imaging (mammography and ultrasound) findings, a recommendation for biopsy can be made with more assurance.

Because malignant lesions can masquerade as benign and vice versa, there can be overlap in the imaging characteristics of benign and malignant lesions. Because there is overlap, the most definitive method of differentiation between benign and malignant is, of course, biopsy, which should be performed for any suspicious finding. This article addresses the features that help the reader to determine what is suspicious as well as features of a few classic benign entities on MR imaging.

Breast MR imaging technique

The ability to characterize lesions is extremely dependent on the chosen technique. If one choses a low spatial resolution protocol, one loses much information about shape and border characteristics as well as internal enhancement. If one choses a low temporal resolution technique, valuable kinetic information about how the lesion enhances is lost. Therefore, it is important to choose a technique that allows high spatial as well as temporal resolution.

There is no "gold standard" technique for performing breast MR imaging. Many techniques are available and widely used depending on hardware and software capabilities and personal preferences. Bilateral examination should be performed. Most investigators use a fat-suppressed T1-weighted sequence and obtain images before and after gadolinium-diethylenetriamine penta-acetic acid (DTPA) administration. Each series should be performed in less than 2 minutes, and at least three postcontrast series should be obtained. High spatial resolution techniques favor lesion morphologic analysis, and rapid acquisition is used for assessing enhancement profiles. A bright fluid sequence (T2-weighted sequence or short tau inversion recovery [STIR]) is useful for identifying breast cysts, which can be simple or hemorrhagic, in addition to myxoid fibroadenomas and lymph nodes, which can be high in signal intensity (SI) on this sequence.

In addition to providing descriptions of the morphologic and kinetic findings, it is important that the MR imaging report should have a final recommendation (BI-RADS 1–6) to convey the level of suspicion to the referring physician. If a recommendation for biopsy is made (BI-RADS 4 or 5), it should be clearly reported in the final impression and a final assessment category should be specified, as in mammography. The ability to biopsy under MR imaging or to refer the patient to a center that performs MR imaging–guided biopsy is essential.

Breast histopathology and MR imaging

Breast disease is superbly seen and delineated by using breast MR imaging. To allow identification and characterization of small lesions, slice thickness should be 2 to 3 mm or less so that volume averaging is not an issue. Because breast cancer can grow along a duct system extending from the terminal duct lobular unit into the breast as an invasive mass or extending along the duct system in a segmental fashion to the nipple, breast MR imaging is exquisitely poised to depict the spread of disease as long as there is increased vascularity associated with the disease. For this reason, sagittal and axial display is preferred to coronal display. Three-dimensional maximum intensity projection (MIP) reconstructions can nicely demonstrate such ductal enhancement patterns (Fig. 1).

A basic understanding of cancer growth and spread in the breast aids in the analysis of the morphologic features seen with breast MR imaging. Similarly, knowledge of the histopathology of benign lesions, such as the different types of fibroadenomas, can aid in the interpretation of benign findings. For example, a slowly enhancing mass may represent a sclerotic hyalinized fibroadenoma, whereas a rapidly enhancing mass may represent a myxoid fibroadenoma. Fibroadenomas may also contain fibrous nonenhancing bands; if these are identified, a benign diagnosis can be made comfortably.

Background enhancement

Because breast fibroglandular tissue has associated vessels, there can be enhancement of the background parenchyma after contrast administration. This is not pathologic enhancement but rather normal variant enhancement. The degree that the background enhances varies on the basis of the individual as well as on the time that the patient is imaged in the menstrual cycle (applies only to premenopausal women). Because background enhancement can obscure lesions and make interpretation more difficult, it is helpful to classify the level of background enhancement as minimal (Fig. 2), moderate (Fig. 3), or marked (Fig. 4). In a way, this background enhancement description is analogous to density on mammography. It is well known that cancers may not be detected in a dense mammogram. Similarly, on MR imaging, cancers may be missed on MR imaging with marked background enhancement. It gives an idea of the level of confidence of finding an abnormality and the likelihood that one may be not imaged.

Description of morphologic features

Morphologic analysis is best performed with high spatial resolution techniques that allow evaluation

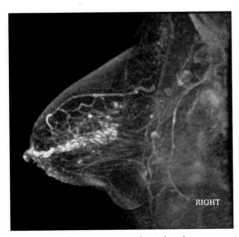

Fig. 1. MIP demonstrates ductal enhancement.

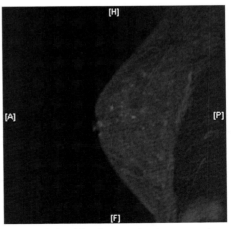

Fig. 2. Minimal background enhancement.

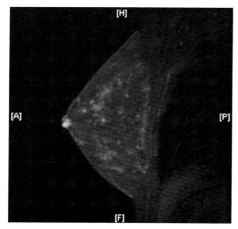

Fig. 3. Moderate background enhancement.

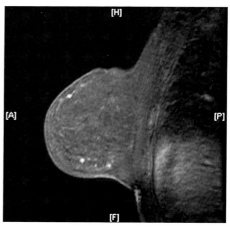

Fig. 5. Focus.

of the mass shape and border so that suspicious spiculated masses can be differentiated from round benign-appearing masses. Also, with high spatial resolution, the borders and internal architecture of the lesion can be assessed and the pattern of enhancement can be readily characterized.

Focus

A focus is a tiny punctate dot of enhancement that is nonspecific and too small to be characterized. A focus is generally less than 5 mm in size. A focus is clearly not a space-occupying lesion or mass (Fig. 5). Multiple foci create a stippled pattern of enhancement (Fig. 6).

Mass

An enhancing lesion on MR imaging can be described as a mass if it displaces tissue and has space-occupying properties. A mass is generally greater than 5 mm in size (Fig. 7).

Shape and margins

The shape and margins of masses can be described. Mass shape can be described as round, oval, lobulated, or irregular. Margins of masses are smooth, irregular, or spiculated. Spiculated or irregular masses (Fig. 8) are suspicious for carcinoma, whereas a smooth margin is more suggestive of a benign lesion. It is important to realize that margin analysis is dependent on spatial resolution and that even irregular borders can appear relatively smooth when insufficient resolution is used. Therefore, carcinoma may present with benign imaging features on MR imaging, particularly when small in size. In general, margin and shape analysis should be performed on the first postcontrast image to avoid wash-out and progressive enhancement of the surrounding breast tissue, which could obscure lesion analysis.

Internal enhancement

Internal enhancement of masses can be described as homogeneous, heterogeneous, rim, dark internal

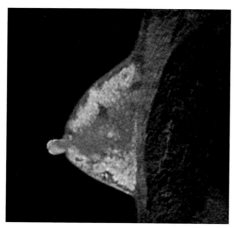

Fig. 4. Marked background enhancement.

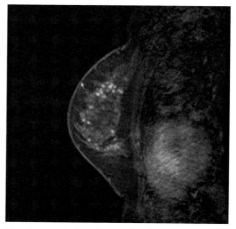

Fig. 6. Stippled pattern of enhancement.

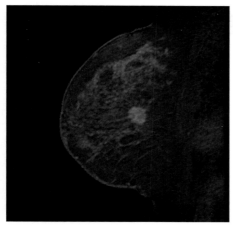

Fig. 7. Mass.

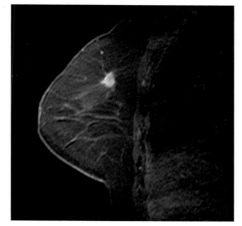

Fig. 9. Homogeneous internal enhancement.

septation, enhancing internal septation, and central enhancement. Homogeneous enhancement is confluent and uniform (Fig. 9). Heterogeneous enhancement is nonuniform with areas of variable SI (Fig. 10).

Homogeneous enhancement is suggestive of a benign process; however, in small lesions, one must be careful, because spatial resolution may limit evaluation. For this reason, kinetics evaluation plays an important role in the evaluation of small, round, smooth, homogeneous masses. If kinetics show wash-out, the lesion becomes much more suspicious. Heterogeneous enhancement is more characteristic of malignant lesions, especially if rim enhancement is present (Fig. 11). Enhancing internal septations (Fig. 12) and central enhancement (Fig. 13) are suspicious for malignancy.

Nonenhancing internal septations are classic for fibroadenomas, although only 40% demonstrate this finding [5]. When nonenhancing internal septations are present, these masses can be considered

benign with a high degree of certainty (>95% according to Nunes and colleagues [6]) (Fig. 14). Similarly, nonenhancing masses are also likely benign fibroadenomas that have a high hyaline content (Fig. 15). Other benign lesions include an inflammatory cyst that enhances peripherally (Fig. 16) and benign fat necrosis (Fig. 17) that exhibits rim enhancement with central low signal indicating fatty content. These latter two lesions should be recognized as potential pitfalls in interpretation of "rim"-enhancing lesions. The cyst can generally be identified on a T2-weighted image, and fat necrosis can often be recognized based on the patient's history and mammographic findings and any non–fat-suppressed images, if performed.

Nonmass enhancement

If the enhancement is neither a focus nor a mass, it is classified as non–mass-like enhancement. Non–mass-like enhancement is classified according to the distribution of the enhancement and can be

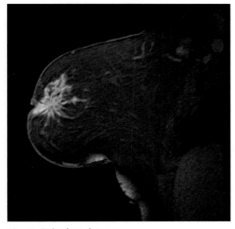

Fig. 8. Spiculated mass.

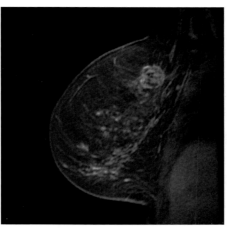

Fig. 10. Heterogeneous internal enhancement.

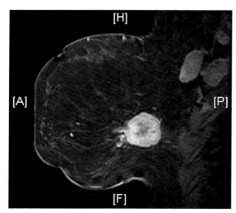

Fig. 11. Rim enhancement.

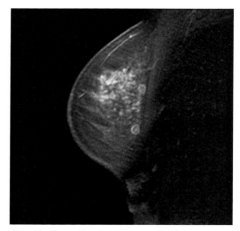

Fig. 13. Central enhancement.

described as focal area, linear, ductal, segmental, regional, multiple regions, or diffuse. Linear enhancement is enhancement in a line. Ductal enhancement may also be linear but would correspond to one or more ducts in orientation and is suspicious for ductal carcinoma in situ (DCIS). Segmental refers to enhancement that is triangular in shape with the apex at the nipple and is suspicious for DCIS within a single branching duct system (Fig. 18). Regional enhancement is enhancement that does not correspond to a single duct system; however, it may be within multiple ducts.

Linear enhancement can be further described as smooth or clumped. As with smooth masses, smooth linear enhancement is suggestive of a benign process. Irregular enhancement refers to any nonsmooth enhancement and may be continuous or discontinuous (Fig. 19). It is suspicious for malignancy. Clumped enhancement refers to an aggregate of enhancing masses or foci that may be confluent in a cobblestone pattern (Fig. 20). Linear enhancement is suggestive of DCIS, especially if

clumped. Liberman and colleagues [5] reported that ductal enhancement had a positive biopsy rate of 26%. The differential diagnosis of ductal enhancement includes carcinoma (usually DCIS), atypical ductal hyperplasia (ADH), lobular carcinoma in situ (LCIS), and benign findings such as fibrocystic change, ductal hyperplasia, and fibrosis.

Segmental, regional, or diffuse enhancement can be further described as homogeneous, heterogeneous, stippled/punctate, clumped, or reticular/dendritic. Stippled refers to multiple and often innumerable punctate foci that are approximately 1 to 2 mm in size and appear scattered throughout an area of the breast that does not usually conform to a duct system (Fig. 21). Stippled enhancement is characteristic of benign normal variant parenchymal enhancement or fibrocystic changes. Regional enhancement and diffuse enhancement are more characteristic of benign disease, such as proliferative changes (Fig. 22), although multicentric DCIS may have this appearance (Fig. 23).

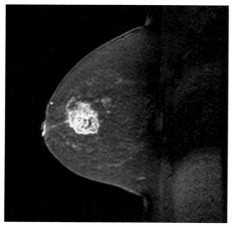

Fig. 12. Enhancing internal septations.

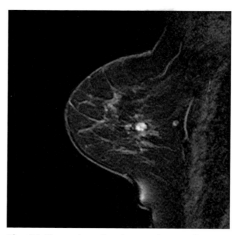

Fig. 14. Nonenhancing internal septations.

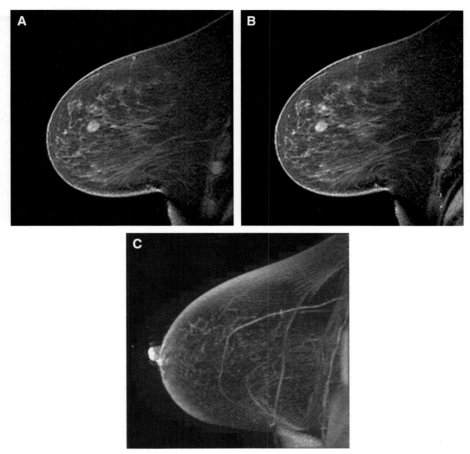

Fig. 15. Nonenhancing mass: precontrast (*A*) postcontrast (*B*), and MIP subtraction (*C*).

Schnall and coworkers [2,7] reported that the probability of cancer was highest using a descriptor of focal mass (63% malignant), followed by ductal enhancement (59% malignant). Area enhancement and patchy enhancement each had a probability of cancer of approximately 50%.

Description of kinetic features

Enhancement kinetics are particularly helpful if the lesion has a benign morphologic appearance. Any suspicious morphologic feature (eg, rim enhancement, spiculated margins) should prompt a biopsy;

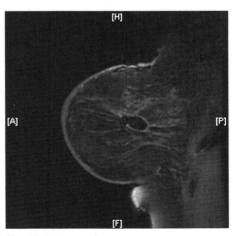

Fig. 16. Inflammatory cyst.

Fig. 17. Fat necrosis.

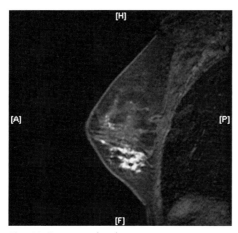

Fig. 18. Segmental enhancement.

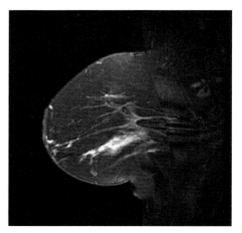

Fig. 20. Clumped enhancement.

therefore, kinetic analysis in these cases, although interesting, is not necessary, because the decision to perform a biopsy has already been made. In the case of a well-defined mass that could quite possibly be benign, however, enhancement kinetic data may help one to decide whether a biopsy is required or whether it is safe to recommend follow-up of the lesion.

To perform kinetic analysis, high temporal resolution is required so that multiple acquisitions can be obtained after the intravenous contrast bolus. In general, the time per sequential acquisition should be less than 2 minutes. If breast MR imaging is performed in this manner, spatial resolution need not be sacrificed. Because there may be a trade-off between spatial and temporal resolution, an extremely rapid sequence that would provide excellent temporal resolution resulting in excellent dynamic data may be compromised with respect to the morphologic information

about the lesion. Newer sequences, usually those using parallel imaging techniques, allow simultaneous bilateral imaging with high temporal and spatial resolution so that no compromise need be made.

Kinetic techniques analyze the enhancement rate of a lesion by manually placing a region of interest (ROI) over the most intensely enhancing area of the lesion. More recently, computer-aided detection (CAD) systems are available to assist in the generation of curves and can also provide angiogenesis maps that demonstrate the dynamic characteristics of lesions. The SI in the ROI is then plotted over time. Clearly, the more acquisitions obtained after intravenous contrast administration, the more points there are on the curve. Additionally, the faster the acquisition, the more potential information is obtained about the curve. If multiple ROIs are placed, the most suspicious curve should be reported. The ROI size should be greater than three

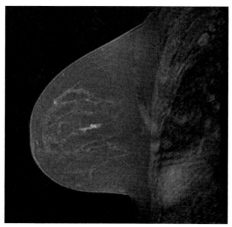

Fig. 19. Linear irregular enhancement.

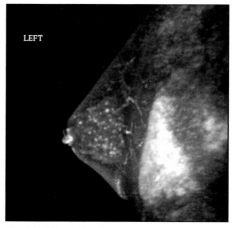

Fig. 21. Stippled enhancement.

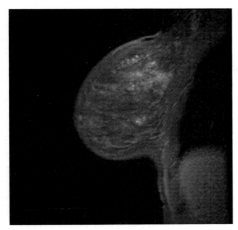

Fig. 22. Regional enhancement.

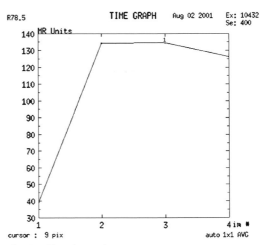

Fig. 24. Time intensity curve.

pixels. SI increase is measured relative to the baseline SI value:

$$\left[(SI_{post} - SI_{pre})/SI_{pre}\right] \times 100\%$$

where SI_{pre} is the baseline SI and SI_{post} is the SI after contrast injection [8].

Kinetic techniques generate time/signal intensity curves (TICs) (Fig. 24). The information derived from these curves can be interpreted in several ways. There is fair consensus that the most important features of the curve involve the initial enhancement phase and the delayed enhancement phase. A rapid initial enhancement and a delayed wash-out enhancement are suspicious.

Kuhl and colleagues [9] described three general types of curves that rely less on the absolute value of the enhancement than on the shape of the enhancement curve. A type I curve is continuous enhancement increasing with time. A type II curve reaches a plateau phase, where maximum SI is reached approximately 2 to 3 minutes after

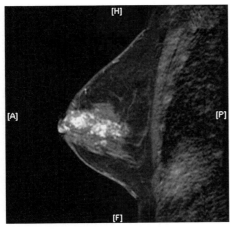

Fig. 23. Multicentric DCIS.

injection and the SI remains constant at this level. Type III is a wash-out curve, where there has been a decrease in SI after peak enhancement has been reached within 2 to 3 minutes.

As a general rule, benign lesions follow a type I curve and malignant lesions follow a type III curve. A type II curve can be seen with benign and malignant lesions. As with morphologic analysis, malignant lesions can exhibit benign kinetics and vice versa. Kuhl and colleagues [9] showed that 57% of malignant lesions demonstrated a type III curve and 83% of benign lesions showed a type I or II curve.

Predictive morphologic features

Benign disease

Certain specific morphologic features can be predictive of benign disease. Nunes and coworkers [6,10,11] reported that certain MR imaging findings are predictive of benign disease, such as smooth or lobulated borders (97%–100% negative predictive value [NPV] for malignancy), absence of lesion enhancement (100% NPV), enhancement less than surrounding breast stroma (93%–100% NPV), and absence of a lesion (92% NPV). The presence of nonenhancing internal septations in a smooth or lobulated mass is highly specific for the diagnosis of fibroadenoma (93%–97% specificity). A stippled pattern of enhancement is predictive of benign fibrocystic changes.

Malignant disease

Certain morphologic characteristics are suggestive of malignancy. Findings that are highly predictive of malignant disease include spiculated margins (76%–88% positive predictive value [PPV]) and rim enhancement (79%–92% PPV) (Box 2; Table 1) [5–7].

The strongest correlations that Nunes and co-workers [6,10,11] found between lesion appearance and pathologic findings were smooth mass and fibrocystic change, lobulated mass with nonenhancing internal septations and fibroadenoma, enhancing irregular or spiculated mass and invasive ductal carcinoma, spiculated mass and invasive tubular carcinoma or radial scar, enhancing lobulated mass and medullary or colloid carcinoma, ductal enhancement and DCIS, and regional enhancement and DCIS.

Suggested algorithm for interpretation

An approach to breast MR imaging interpretation is outlined in this section. Initial evaluation of T2-weighted images is performed to determine if high-signal masses, such as cysts, lymph nodes, or myxoid fibroadenomas, are present. Evaluation of the nonenhanced T1-weighted images documents the presence of high-signal hemorrhagic or protein-aceous cysts as well as high signal within dilated ducts. The postcontrast T1-weighted images demonstrate the presence of any enhancing masses or non–mass-like areas of enhancement. Morphologic analysis of the architectural features of a mass would then determine if the margins are irregular or spiculated, findings that would be highly

suggestive of malignancy. At this point, a biopsy would be recommended. A search for the mass by ultrasound may be helpful to allow percutaneous biopsy.

If the mass demonstrates smooth margins and rim enhancement, because rim enhancement is highly predictive of malignancy, a biopsy would be recommended in this case as well, once the false-positive causes of rim enhancement, such as inflamed cyst and fat necrosis, have been excluded. Similarly, ductal enhancement that is irregular or clumped is suspicious for DCIS, and a biopsy generally results from this finding.

If the mass is homogeneously enhancing, however, and demonstrates smooth borders, possibly representing a benign finding, kinetic analysis can be extremely helpful. Kinetics can determine whether this is indeed likely benign (type I curve) or possibly malignant (type II or III curve), prompting a biopsy. Because a homogeneously enhancing smooth mass with a type I curve has been reported in some malignant lesions, short-term follow up in 6 months may be advisable if this combination of findings is found to document benignity. There are few published reports to validate 6 months of follow-up in the setting of MR imaging; however, because this population undergoing MR imaging is at elevated risk, it is likely that the malignancy rate for 6 months of follow-up for probably benign MR imaging findings is greater than the less than accepted 2% rate for mammography.

For areas of non–mass-like enhancement, kinetic analysis may be helpful, because findings, such as regional enhancement, can be found in benign and malignant breast pathologic conditions, such as proliferative changes and DCIS. Kinetic curves may have little use in stippled enhancement, because the tiny foci of enhancement are likely too small for accurate placement of an ROI. Similarly, kinetic curves are not useful for DCIS. Evaluation of DCIS is usually based entirely on morphologic criteria (which is why DCIS may have been missed for many years by investigators relying solely on kinetic evaluation for biopsy).

Summary

The ACR BI-RADS MRI lexicon incorporates morphologic and kinetic features of lesions identified on breast MR imaging. This brief article is aimed at introducing this material and should not be used as a definitive guide. Because the breast MR imaging lexicon is a work in progress, there are many areas that need exploring and better characterization. It is hoped that the radiologist uses the terms and concepts presented here as a template to which future lexicon terminology can be added.

Table 1:   Positive predictive value for malignancy

Descriptor	PPV
Ductal enhancement	80%
Regional enhancement	58%
Irregular focal mass	81%
Spiculated mass	88%
Rim enhancement	79%

Data from Refs. [5–7].

References

[1] Technical report of the International Working Group on Breast MRI. J Magn Reson Imaging 1999;10:978–1015.

[2] Schnall MD, Ikeda DM. Lesion diagnosis working group report. J Magn Reson Imaging 1999; 10:982–90.

[3] Ikeda DM, Baker DR, Daniel BL. Magnetic resonance imaging of breast cancer: clinical indications and breast MRI reporting system. J Magn Reson Imaging 2000;12(6):975–83.

[4] American College of Radiology. Breast imaging reporting and data system (BI-RADS). 3rd edition. Reston (VA): American College of Radiology; 1998.

[5] Liberman L, Morris EA, Dershaw DD, et al. Ductal enhancement on MR imaging of the breast. AJR Am J Roentgenol 2003;181:519–25.

[6] Nunes LW, Schnall MD, Siegelman ES, et al. Diagnostic performance characteristics of architectural features revealed by high spatial-resolution MR imaging of the breast. AJR Am J Roentgenol 1997;169:409–15.

[7] Schnall MD, Blume J, Bluemke DA, et al. Diagnostic and architectural features at breast MR imaging: multicenter study. Radiology 2006;238: 42–53.

[8] Kuhl CK, Schild HH. Dynamic image interpretation of MRI of the breast. J Magn Reson Imaging 2000;12(6):965–74.

[9] Kuhl CK, Mielcareck P, Klaschik S, et al. Dynamic breast MR imaging: are signal intensity time course data useful for differential diagnosis of enhancing lesions? Radiology 1999;211: 101–10.

[10] Nunes LW, Schnall MD, Orel SG, et al. Breast MR imaging: interpretation model. Radiology 1997; 202:833–41.

[11] Nunes LW, Schnall MD, Orel SG, et al. Correlation of lesion appearance and histologic findings for the nodes of a breast MR imaging interpretation model. Radiographics 1999;19: 79–92.

MAGNETIC
RESONANCE
IMAGING CLINICS

Magn Reson Imaging Clin N Am 14 (2006) 305–328

Concepts for Differential Diagnosis in Breast MR Imaging

Christiane K. Kuhl, MD

- Technical groundwork
- Diagnostic criteria for contrast-enhanced breast MR imaging
  Analysis of lesion morphology
  Kinetic curve assessment
  Analysis of lesion signal intensity in precontrast T1-weighted and T2-weighted turbo spin echo images
- MR imaging findings in benign and malignant breast lesions
  Invasive breast cancers
  Intraductal cancers (ductal carcinoma in situ)

- *Lobular carcinoma in situ*
  Breast MR imaging features of benign tumors: fibroadenomas
  Nodular mastopathic changes and focal adenosis
  Hormonal stimulation
  Cysts
  Postsurgical scar
  Fat necrosis
  Radial scar (complex sclerosing lesion)
  Intramammary lymph nodes
  Mastitis
- Suggested readings
- References

Technical groundwork

Probably because of their angiogenic activity, malignant lesions tend to exhibit an increased vessel density and an increased vessel wall permeability compared with normal fibroglandular breast tissue [1,2]. This gives rise to an increased inflow and an accelerated extravasation of an MR imaging contrast agent bolus, thereby causing a signal intensity increase in T1-weighted MR images. Early work on breast MR imaging exploited these effects to enable breast cancer diagnosis in contrast-enhanced MR imaging. To track the fast signal intensity changes that occur after bolus injection of a contrast agent, a so-called "dynamic series" was obtained [3,4]. This consisted of a series of (typically approximately 10) identical T1-weighted gradient echo pulse sequences that were acquired once before and several times after contrast agent injection.

Breast cancer was then diagnosed by comparing pre- and postcontrast images. If a significant signal intensity increase was observed on the first postcontrast acquisition, it was called suspicious, because the assumption was that only (or predominantly) malignant tissues are sufficiently vascularized to produce such early and strong enhancement. The signal intensity increase was considered significant if the signal intensity doubled (ie, rose by 100% after versus before contrast). This or similar thresholds were propagated to be used for differential diagnosis in dynamic contrast-enhanced breast MR imaging. In fact, early publications suggested a high sensitivity and specificity for dynamic breast MR imaging with an enhancement threshold or even only the presence or absence of enhancement as a solitary criterion of differential diagnosis [3–5]. As one would expect, however, there are a wide variety of benign lesions exhibiting enhancement and

Department of Radiology, University of Bonn, Sigmund-Freud-Strasse 25, D-53105 Bonn, Germany
E-mail address: kuhl@uni-bonn.de

doi:10.1016/j.mric.2006.07.002

even many benign lesions exhibiting fast and strong enhancement that would surpass any given threshold. In addition, there are malignant tissues that do not exhibit angiogenic activity that would be sufficient to cause doubled signal intensity after contrast injection. Although it rapidly became obvious that neither enhancement per se nor an enhancement beyond a certain threshold is sufficient for differential diagnosis in breast MR imaging, this concept has survived to the present time and is still in use. The reason for the attractiveness of this concept is its intriguing simplicity: everybody, even somebody without any experience in breast MR imaging, is able to distinguish enhancing from nonenhancing tissue or is able to apply a threshold, such that this concept seems to be an easy and fool-proof way to establish a diagnosis.

From early on, there were two entirely different approaches to breast MR imaging that used different imaging techniques and different diagnostic criteria. The difference was probably just secondary to the fact that there were bilateral breast coils available from European MR imaging vendors, whereas only unilateral coils were available from US system vendors. Consequently, in Europe, bilateral, axial, dynamic, subtracted breast MR imaging was popular, whereas in the United States, unilateral, sagittal, nondynamic, actively fat-suppressed breast MR imaging was propagated.

The reason for this dichotomy of breast MR imaging strategies was the fact that when breast MR imaging was inaugurated in the late 1980s and early 1990s, the performance of MR imaging systems was poor compared with current standards. At that time, fast imaging (with fast being considered an acquisition time of approximately 60 seconds) was only possible with a low in-plane and even lower through-plane image resolution. On the other end of the spectrum, what was called high spatial resolution at that time required long acquisition times, precluding any type of kinetic assessment.

In the early days of breast MR imaging, a so-called "dynamic study" would consist of approximately 11 to 15 sections of a gradient echo pulse sequence that was obtained with a reduced 256 imaging matrix, with a resulting voxel size of 1.5 mm $\times$ 2.5 mm $\times$ 5.0 mm (ie, 18.75 mm^3). The lower the spatial resolution, however, the less readers are inclined to find morphologic criteria for image interpretation useful, such that for differential diagnosis, users of the so-called "dynamic school" in the old days had to rely almost entirely on lesion enhancement kinetics. In turn, if readers used nondynamic imaging with high spatial resolution (with voxel sizes typically ranging around 1.0 mm $\times$ 1.5 mm $\times$ 4 mm [ie, 6 mm^3]), readers would not be able to appreciate the diagnostic information that

is inherent to a kinetic analysis. Thus, there was little, if any, overlap regarding the acquisition parameters or the interpretation criteria that were used for analyzing European or US breast MR imaging studies.

Today, the two schools have greatly merged. It is now possible to acquire high in- and through-plane spatial resolution in a dynamic mode [6]. With current state-of-the-art equipment, bilateral subtracted MR imaging is achievable with approximately 30 sections and a voxel size of 0.6 mm $\times$ 0.6 mm $\times$ 3.0 mm (ie, 1.08 mm^3). In turn, bilateral, sagittal, actively fat-suppressed imaging in a dynamic mode has become available. Accordingly, the principles and diagnostic criteria of the European approach and the US approach can now be integrated instead of compromising on the basis of spatial or temporal resolution. This helps one to exploit the full potential of breast MR imaging and helps to improve the sensitivity and specificity of breast MR imaging compared with the old purely dynamic or purely morphologic approach.

In fact, if one uses such a high spatial resolution, dynamic acquisition breast MR imaging is able to provide diagnostic information that is not delivered by any other breast imaging modality. Unlike mammography and breast ultrasound, contrast-enhanced MR imaging of the breast not only offers information on cross-sectional morphology of lesions but provides information on functional criteria, such as tissue perfusion and capillary permeability, as well as on tissue signal intensities in T1- and T2-weighted pulse sequences. All this can, and should, be evaluated before a final diagnosis is established. In addition, more sophisticated MR imaging techniques are on the horizon that should allow even more detailed tissue analysis. These techniques include magnetic resonance spectroscopy, elastography, and molecular imaging of selective cellular surface targets.

Diagnostic criteria for contrast-enhanced breast MR imaging

In the following section, a systematic approach for image analysis in breast MR imaging is presented, and typical MR imaging findings in benign and malignant breast diseases are listed. To start with, however, it is important to realize that none of the imaging findings mentioned here provides 100% sensitivity or specificity. Accordingly, in each case, the MR imaging findings have to be weighed against the findings made by clinical breast examination, mammography, and breast ultrasound. It is always important to collect all information that is available on the patient before a final diagnosis is established. Breast MR imaging studies should not be interpreted in a vacuum. It is vital to have the respective mammograms available (not only the report but the mammograms themselves) to integrate this information into the final MR imaging report. In addition, the respective patient's clinical findings and her personal or family history have to be considered before a management recommendation is given. One should also keep in mind that a core biopsy is a safe and cost-effective way to clarify suspicious lesions definitively. With the increasing availability of MR imaging–compatible biopsy systems, this also holds true for lesions that are visible by breast MR imaging alone [7–9].

In accordance with the new MR imaging Breast Imaging and Reporting Data System (BI-RADS) lexicon [9,10], diagnostic criteria that are in use for differential diagnosis can be divided into those related to lesion morphology (A), those related to lesion enhancement kinetics (B), and (as an add-on to the BI-RADS lexicon) those related to a lesion's signal intensity in non–fat-suppressed, nonsubtracted, precontrast, T1-weighted and T2-weighted images (C). Because the evaluation of morphologic features is usually based on analysis of postcontrast (subtracted or fat-suppressed) images of enhancing areas, this distinction is somewhat arbitrary. Still, when reading breast MR imaging studies, a step-by-step analysis of the different features is recommended.

When interpreting breast MR imaging studies, the first step is to determine whether there is (1) a mass (Fig. 1), (2) non–mass-like enhancement (Fig. 2), or (3) a focus (Fig. 3).

A focus is an enhancing spot that is less than 5 mm in size (ie, a lesion too small to characterize). This is different for masses and non–mass-like enhancement. The diagnostic pathway ends here; further management depends on the entire clinical picture (eg, presence or absence of breast cancer in the same breast, history of breast cancer, antihormonal medication) rather than on a further analysis of lesion features.

This is different for masses and non–mass-like enhancement. These types are subjected to a careful analysis of morphology, enhancement kinetics, and signal intensity pattern in T1- and T2-weighted images.

In a mass, the differential diagnostic consideration is invasive breast cancer or a benign solid tumor (eg, fibroadenoma). In non–mass-like enhancement, the differential diagnosis is between intraductal tumor and mastopathic changes (focal adenosis), hormonal stimulation, inflammatory changes/mastitis, and, rarely, diffusely infiltrating cancer (eg, invasive lobular cancer).

The decision between mass and non–mass-like enhancement initiates two separate diagnostic pathways that require different diagnostic criteria for the further distinction of benign and malignant masses or non–mass-like lesions. Although shape and margins are assessed in masses, in non–mass-like enhancement, this is not done. Instead, its distribution is assessed, with major emphasis on whether or not the enhancement is oriented along the distribution of the milk ducts or not. Analysis of time course kinetics is mainly useful for the differential diagnosis of masses, whereas it is rarely useful for the further classification of non–mass-like enhancement.

Analysis of lesion morphology

Shape and margins

In masses, shape and borders are described with descriptors that are similar to those used for mammography (with the notable exclusion of the term *obscured*, because MR imaging delivers cross-sectional images). The diagnostic implications are quite comparable to the mammographic descriptors. The overall shape is described as round, oval, or irregular; margins are characterized as smooth, lobular, irregular, or spiculated. Of course, an irregular shape and irregular or spiculated margins are more suspicious than an oval mass with smooth borders; everything that holds true for morphologic analysis of shape and margins in mammography also holds true for breast MR imaging.

Distribution

In non–mass-like enhancement, shape and borders are not assessable. Instead, distribution is rated with descriptors that are relatively similar to those used for describing the distribution of grouped calcifications on a mammogram and with similar diagnostic implications. The distribution can follow the ductal system; in this case, it is referred to as being segmental or ductal. Just as mammographic calcifications in segmental or ductal distribution, segmental or ductal enhancement in MR imaging suggests the presence of an intraductal pathologic finding, be it a small ductal carcinoma in situ (DCIS) or papilloma (in ductal enhancement) or a large DCIS or peripheral papillomatosis (in segmental enhancement). If the distribution does not follow the ductal system, it is referred to as linear (a line that does not follow a duct), a focal area (non–mass-like enhancement of less than one quarter of a quadrant), regional enhancement (geographic enhancement of a larger area), enhancement in multiple regions, or diffuse enhancement (confluent enhancement of more or less the entire breast). The finding of multiple regions or diffuse enhancement has approximately the same diagnostic implication as a mammogram with diffuse or scattered calcifications. The probability is high

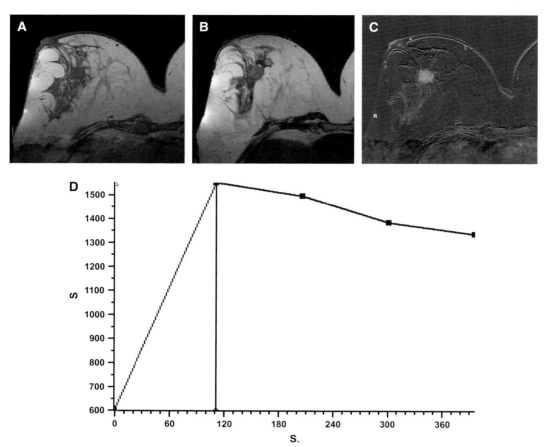

Fig. 1. Enhancing "mass". 48-year-old patient with ductal invasive breast cancer. (*A*) Precontrast, T1-weighted, gradient echo image. (*B*) T2-weighted non-fat suppressed image. (*C*) Post-contrast subtracted image. (*D*) Time/signal intensity diagram. Note the space-occupying mass lesion, which appears to be spherically shaped. (*A, C*) Note the correlate on precontrast T1-weighted and T2-weighted TSE images. (*A, B*) The mass exhibits typical features of breast cancer, including morphology and kinetics (wash-out).

that all calcification (all enhancement in MR imaging) is attributable to microcystic blunt duct disease (adenosis in MR imaging); however, it is impossible to determine definitively whether any given small calcification (area of enhancement in MR imaging) may be attributable to DCIS or a small invasive cancer.

Although ductal, segmental, regional or diffuse enhancement in MR imaging is approximately equivalent to the mammographic findings of calcifications in ductal, segmental, regional, or diffuse distribution, this analogy does not work for the other descriptors of non–mass-like enhancement. A focal area of enhancement or regional enhancement is by no means comparable to the diagnostic implication of a group of calcifications; this is where the analogy fails. A region of enhancement is more often caused by benign changes than by malignant lesions.

If an MR imaging study covers both breasts (which is highly desirable and is the case in all axial, dynamic, contrast-enhanced techniques), it is possible to compare both breasts and decide whether a non–mass-enhancing area is symmetric or not. Obviously, bilateral symmetric non–mass-like enhancement in any distribution is more often caused by benign changes than by malignant lesions. Accordingly, side-by-side comparisons in bilateral studies are helpful to deal with the most frequent cause of benign non–mass-like enhancement (ie, adenosis [ductal or lobular hyperplasia] or hormonal stimulation).

Internal enhancement
As an add-on compared with mammography and breast ultrasound, lesion internal enhancement (internal architecture) is described. Some of the most powerful diagnostic criteria for the differentiation

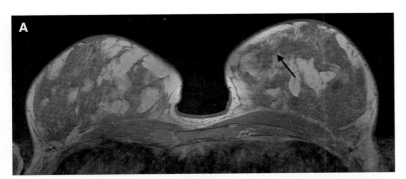

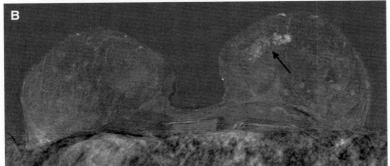

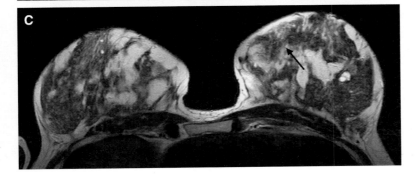

Fig. 2. Non–mass-like enhancement in a 43-year-old patient with DCIS. (*A*) Precontrast, T1-weighted, gradient echo image. (*B*) Postcontrast subtracted image. (*C*) T2-weighted non–fat-suppressed image. Note that the area of enhancement has no space-occupying effects. There seems to be normal fibroglandular tissue at the site of enhancement (*arrows*). Note the segmental distribution, following the milk ducts. Note the clumped internal architecture.

of benign and malignant tumors belong to this category. Internal enhancement can be homogeneous or heterogeneous or can affect only the periphery of a lesion (rim enhancement). Finally, bright (enhancing) or dark internal septations may be identified. Although homogeneous enhancement is usually found in benign masses, rim enhancement or enhancing internal septations are highly suggestive of malignancy. In turn, dark septations (if present within a lobular or oval mass) are typical of fibroadenomas. Heterogeneous enhancement can be seen in invasive breast cancers and in partly sclerotic fibroadenomas.

Internal enhancement in areas of non–mass-like enhancement is described as being homogeneous, heterogeneous, stippled, or clumped. Although virtually all causes of non–mass-like enhancement (eg, hormonal stimulation of normal breast tissue, adenosis, inflammation/mastitis, DCIS, diffusely infiltrating cancer like lobular cancer) can exhibit all types of internal enhancement, there is evidence that clumped and stippled internal enhancement is more suggestive of DCIS rather than of benign non–mass-like enhancement. The predictive value of these features is, however, much lower than that offered by the finding of dark internal septations or rim enhancement in masses.

Kinetic curve assessment

Kinetic analysis is mainly useful to differentiate masses that exhibit rapid or medium enhancement further. It is not useful to classify masses with slow enhancement further, and it is rarely useful in non–mass-like enhancement. The reason is that kinetic criteria are unreliable for the diagnosis of DCIS or diffusely infiltrating lobular cancer, which are the two most important differential diagnoses in non–mass-like enhancement. In a focus, no further

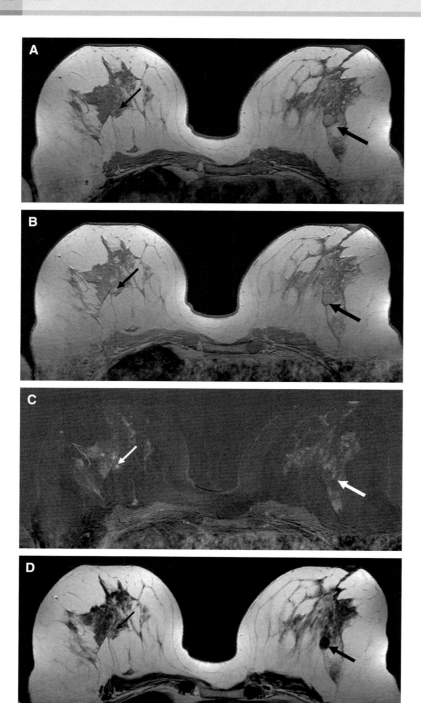

Fig. 3. An enhancing focus and a proteinaceous cyst. 42-year-old-patient with adenosis and fibrocystic changes. (*A*) Precontrast, T1-weighted, gradient echo image. (*B*) Postcontrast image. (*C*) Postcontrast subtracted image. (*D*) T2-weighted non–fat-suppressed image. Note that the enhancing lesion (*thin arrows*) is too small to characterize shape, margins, or internal architecture. Note the proteinaceous cyst in the left breast (*thick arrows*) with bright signal precontrast (*A*), extremely dark signal on the T2-weighted TSE image (*D*), and no enhancement (*C*).

kinetic analysis is done, just as no further assessment of morphologic details is performed.

For analysis of enhancement kinetics, we look at how fast a signal intensity increase appears in a lesion after contrast injection (early rise or wash-in rates), how strong the signal intensity increase is with respect to baseline (precontrast) lesion signal intensity, and what happens with the signal after the early postcontrast phase (delayed-phase enhancement). To evaluate kinetics, a small region of interest (ROI) is placed selectively in the part of an enhancing area that appears brightest on the first postcontrast image. Although computer-assisted detection (CAD) software may facilitate this by color-coding the degree or type of enhancement in a given lesion and may assist in interpreting breast MR imaging studies, CAD users may be tempted to overemphasize kinetic aspects of breast MR imaging differential diagnosis by simply calling all areas marked by the CAD system and disregarding others that are not marked. Moreover, CAD systems tend to use a fixed enhancement threshold or wash-out threshold for differential diagnosis of enhancing lesions, which is clearly inappropriate.

Early rise

Wash-in rates can be quantified and given in percent signal intensity increase. To account for differences in baseline tissue T1 relaxation times, enhancement is calculated as signal intensity increase relative to baseline values Relative signal intensity increase that occurs in a certain period—usually the first postcontrast minute—is referred to as enhancement rate (eg, 80% per minute). We distinguish slow, medium, and rapid early rise. There is no definition as to what exactly constitutes slow versus medium or rapid early enhancement; this has to be defined individually for each setup. The reason is that quantitative enhancement rates may vary with different types of pulse sequences, contrast agent injection modes, site of venous injection, heart rate, and types of equipment. In our setup (1.5-T system, two-dimensional, gradient echo, gadolinium diethylenetriamine penta-acetic acid [Gd-DTPA] at a dose of 0.1 mmol/kg as a bolus via an 18-gauge venous line, followed by a saline flush at a rate of 20 mL), a wash-in rate of more than 80% represents fast enhancement; a 30% signal intensity increase or less is referred to as slow enhancement.

The rationale of calculating enhancement rates is based on the observation that malignant lesions tend to have higher wash-in rates than benign ones. In fact, most invasive breast cancers exhibit fast strong enhancement that peaks in the early postcontrast phase. This is also intuitively used by radiologists who do not use kinetics for lesion differential diagnosis. Also in purely morphologic approaches for interpreting breast MR imaging studies, a lesion appears more conspicuous if it exhibits a bright postcontrast signal, which is the same as strong and rapid wash-in.

Although rapid wash-in during the early postcontrast phase is found in most (approximately 80%) invasive cancers, slowly enhancing invasive cancers do exist; mainly, they belong to the lobular type or exhibit abundant desmoplastic activity. Therefore, if one uses an enhancement threshold, one runs the risk of missing these cancers. In addition, a huge variety of benign lesions exhibit rapid and strong enhancement, such that the use of an enhancement threshold can cause a high number of false-positive findings as well.

Moreover, quantitative enhancement rates vary with different types of equipment. Accordingly, it is impossible to define an enhancement threshold that would be applicable across different setups and vendors. In fact, the use of an enhancement threshold to diagnose breast cancer had been proposed back in the 1990s when dynamic contrast-enhanced breast MR imaging offered such poor spatial resolution that a meaningful analysis of morphologic details was impossible. Since then, MR imaging technology has improved, however, such that it is possible to obtain high spatial resolution and dynamic fast acquisition. With high spatial and high temporal resolution, differential diagnosis criteria have been developed that offer a much better differentiation of benign and malignant lesions than what is offered by using an enhancement threshold alone. With the advent of CAD systems, it seems that the idea of an enhancement threshold celebrates resurrection. This should be discouraged, particularly because enhancement thresholds depend on many confounding factors, and thus may not be copied from one institution to another.

Delayed-phase enhancement

The further fate of the contrast agent is usually assessed visually by looking at the time/signal intensity curves. We distinguish three different types: persistent enhancement (curve exhibits steady signal intensity increase), plateau (fast early upstroke, followed by a plateau after the third postcontrast minute), or wash-out (fast early upstroke, followed by a loss of signal intensity after the third postcontrast minute). The rationale for assessing curve shape is that a persistent time course is indicative of a benign lesion, whereas a wash-out time course supports the diagnosis of a malignant lesion. It is speculated that wash-out is caused by the increased leakage of vessels in malignant lesions. A plateau time course may be found in benign and malignant lesions.

The curve type analysis is done complementary to the morphologic analysis and is mostly useful for differential diagnosis of masses that exhibit fast enhancement. Lesions with medium or slow early rise (ie, lesions with only moderate or poor angiogenic activity) usually exhibit a persistent time course, such that the absence of wash-out cannot be used as a sign of benignity.

Analysis of lesion signal intensity in precontrast T1-weighted and T2-weighted turbo spin echo images

Just as in any other application of MR imaging, tissue signal intensities should be evaluated to help classify enhancing lesions. There is a wealth of diagnostic information inherent to non–fat-suppressed precontrast images that can be used for further differential diagnosis of fat necrosis, intramammary lymph nodes, and inflammatory cysts as well as for the distinction of fibroadenomas and breast cancers. Accordingly, in addition to morphologic and kinetic features, a careful analysis of the lesion's signal intensity in non–fat-suppressed T2-weighted images and precontrast, non–fat-suppressed, T1-weighted images should always be done.

If bright signal is seen within a lesion on non–fat-suppressed, precontrast, T1-weighted images, this is strong evidence for a benign finding. The only exception could be a lesion that underwent a core biopsy with significant hematoma; however, lesions that have undergone a biopsy should not pose diagnostic difficulties anyway, because the histologic findings of the lesion should already be known. If a space-occupying mass appears isointense in a non–fat-suppressed, precontrast, T1-weighted image compared with the adjacent fibroglandular tissue, this should raise the suspicion of breast cancer. If a mass exhibits low signal intensity in the same pulse sequence compared with normal adjacent tissue, this is more suggestive of fibroadenomas.

Moreover, what is known as the halo phenomenon in mammography is also found in breast MR imaging. It is caused by the displaced fatty tissue around a tumor that does not grow invasively but has pushing margins and a clear-cut interface with the fatty tissue. The MR imaging halo can best be appreciated in non–fat-suppressed, precontrast, T1-weighted images, where the displaced fatty tissue is depicted to embrace a well-circumscribed space-occupying mass.

In addition to the T1-weighted dynamic contrast-enhanced series, high spatial resolution, non–fat-suppressed, T2-weighted turbo spin echo (TSE) or fast spin echo (FSE) images are acquired with an anatomic position exactly matching that of the dynamic T1-weighted series. By doing so, an accurate comparison of a lesion's signal intensity in T1-weighted pre- and postcontrast images and its signal intensity in non–fat-suppressed T2-weighted images becomes feasible. Benign masses, such as fibroadenomas or intramammary lymph nodes, usually exhibit a hyperintense signal compared with normal fibroglandular tissue. The typical dark internal septations of myxoid fibroadenomas are sometimes even best visualized in T2-weighted TSE images against the bright myxoid stroma. Most breast cancers exhibit an iso- or hypointense signal compared with regular fibroglandular tissue. This is with the notable exception of mucinous and medullar cancer. Fatty tissue signal (bright on T2- and T1-weighted images) inside a mass is clearly indicative of a benign mass.

Coding breast density

In screening and diagnostic mammography, the parenchymal density is coded according to the American College of Radiology (ACR) categories 1 (fatty breast) through 4 (dense fibroglandular tissue). This is done with the intention to communicate the level of accuracy that can be expected from a given mammogram. The rationale is to indicate that sensitivity and specificity suffer in proportion to breast density and that, for example, in a patient with dense breast tissue, a negative mammogram may not be offering the level of sensitivity that is required to rule out the presence of breast cancer. Based on the current BI-RADS lexicon, breast density in MR imaging is coded by assessing the extent of residual breast tissue. This, however, does not acknowledge the fact that in contrast-enhanced breast MR imaging, it is not the extent of residual breast tissue that would interfere with the diagnosis of breast cancer. Rather, it is the contrast enhancement of the background fibroglandular tissue that determines the interpretability of a breast MR imaging study. Enhancement is by no means determined by the amount of residual fibroglandular tissue. Rather, it is the respective composition (volume of glandular versus connective tissue) and degree of hormonal stimulation that determine the degree of background enhancement. Strong background enhancement that already appears in the early postcontrast phase substantially reduces the sensitivity and specificity of a given breast MR imaging study, much like a radiographically dense breast reduces the sensitivity and specificity of a mammogram, because it may obscure (mask) enhancing invasive cancers and DCIS and may lead to unnecessary biopsies because of enhancing areas. Accordingly, we propose to grade background enhancement instead (or in addition to) the mere amount of the breast tissue, according to the categories of absent, minimal, moderate, and severe, with the implication of a perfect, high, moderately impaired, and severely impaired sensitivity of breast MR imaging (Fig. 4).

MR imaging findings in benign and malignant breast lesions

Invasive breast cancers

The typical invasive breast cancer (Figs. 5 and 6) appears as a mass with an irregular shape and with irregular or spiculated margins. Internal enhancement is heterogeneous or shows rim enhancement.

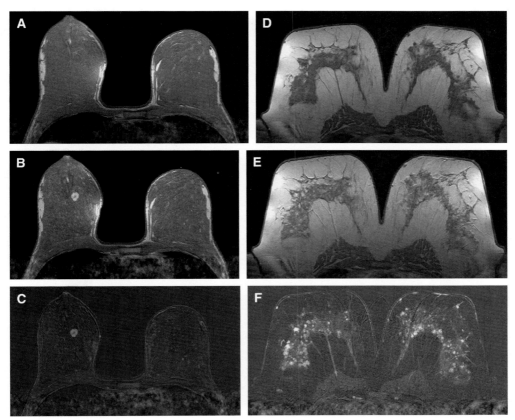

Fig. 4. Coding background enhancement in breast MR imaging (corresponding to ACR coding of breast density in mammograms) (*A–C*) Dense breast tissue (ACR 4) but only minimal background enhancement. (*D–F*) Partly involuted breast (ACR 2 on mammography) but with severe background enhancement in MR imaging, reducing the diagnostic utility of the study. A 42-year-old patient with a palpable lump in the central portion of the right breast. Mammogram reveals dense breast tissue, rated as ACR 4. Precontrast (*A*), postcontrast (*B*), and postcontrast (*C*) subtracted images. At MR imaging, the fibroglandular tissue is dense as well. After administration of contrast, however, there is only minimal enhancement of background fibroglandular tissue, such that the diagnostic utility is not impaired. An enhancing mass is seen with a round shape, smooth borders, central internal septations, and bright signal on a T2-weighted TSE image (not shown). A diagnosis of fibroadenoma was established. Because of the absence of enhancement of the fibroglandular tissue, diagnostic accuracy of breast MR imaging is high. Precontrast (*D*), postcontrast (*E*), and postcontrast (*F*) subtracted images of a 62-year-old patient with biopsy-proven cancer in the left breast at the 12-o'clock position (not shown). Breast MR imaging was performed to rule out multicentric disease. There is multifocal-diffuse early and strong enhancement of the entire background fibroglandular tissue. This is severe background enhancement. Just as in a mammogram with dense breast tissue, additional cancer foci may be masked (or mimicked) by enhancing fibroglandular tissue. The sensitivity and specificity of breast MR imaging are substantially reduced, if not annihilated.

At kinetic analysis, the typical invasive cancer exhibits rapid and strong enhancement, followed by wash-out in the early postcontrast phase. In T1-weighted precontrast images and on non–fat-suppressed T2-weighted images, the typical invasive breast cancer exhibits low signal intensity equivalent to or lower than that of normal fibroglandular tissue.

Depending on the spatial resolution one uses, approximately 10% to 20% of cancers may exhibit smooth margins. With low spatial resolution, spicules may not be resolved, such that breast cancers may appear misleadingly well circumscribed in low spatial resolution studies (ie, studies with an in-plane pixel size of more than 1 mm). If rim enhancement is suspected on postcontrast subtracted or fat-suppressed images, one has to make sure that no pseudo–rim enhancement is caused by a cyst with inflammatory changes or by fresh fat necrosis. Again, this is achievable by analyzing nonsubtracted, non–fat-suppressed, precontrast T1- and T2-weighted images. If the presence of an inflammatory cyst or fat necrosis has been excluded, rim enhancement is such a specific finding that this

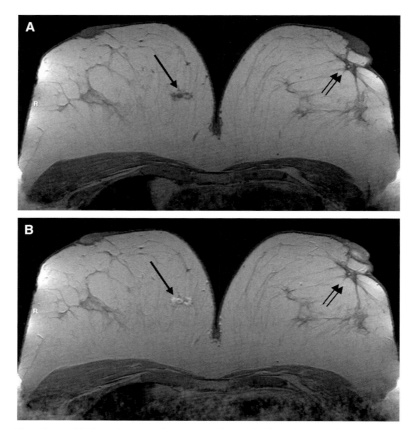

Fig. 5. 53-year-old patient with invasive ductal cancer on her right (*single arrows*) and fat necrosis on her left. There was a history of benign breast biopsy on the left 4 years ago with a scar and central fatty tissue necrosis on the left (*double arrows*). (*A*) Precontrast, T1-weighted, gradient echo image. (*B*) Postcontrast image. (*C*) Postcontrast subtracted image. (*D*) Time/signal intensity curve of the enhancing mass. Note the irregular mass with spiculated margins on the right. Note the heterogeneous internal enhancement in (*C*). Note the rapid early enhancement and wash-out at kinetic analysis in (*D*). Note scar tissue with mass effect on the left (*double arrows*) with central bright signal in (*A*), consistent with fat necrosis. Note that there was no enhancement after contrast injection (*C*).

finding alone is sufficient to recommend a biopsy of an enhancing mass. Strong and early enhancement (beyond a wash-in rate of 80% in our setup) is seen in approximately 80% of invasive breast cancers. A wash-out time course is found in approximately 60% of cancers (see Figs. 1 and 5; Fig. 7), a plateau time course in 30%, and a persistent time course in approximately 10% (Fig. 8).

The predominant breast MR imaging features of invasive breast cancer can vary with the histologic subtype. Although the regular invasive ductal cancer tends to exhibit most of the previously mentioned typical features of invasive breast cancer, this is less often the case in the other more rare subtypes of invasive breast cancers.

Medullar invasive cancer tends to demonstrate a roundish shape with smooth pushing margins and no signs of infiltrating disease on imaging studies as well as on gross pathologic examination; fortunately, medullar cancer makes up only approximately 5% of all breast cancer cases. It is mostly seen in younger individuals; approximately 60% to 66% of patients with medullar breast cancer are younger than 50 years of age. In carriers of the BRCA1 germline mutation, medullar and atypical-medullar breast cancers are encountered much more often; therefore, in individuals with a significant personal or family history of breast cancer, the presence of (medullar) breast cancer should be considered if well-circumscribed fibroadenoma-like tumors are seen on imaging studies. Because MR imaging offers not only shape and margin but kinetic information and information on internal architecture, it has been shown to be useful for distinguishing fibroadenomas or presumably collapsed cysts from

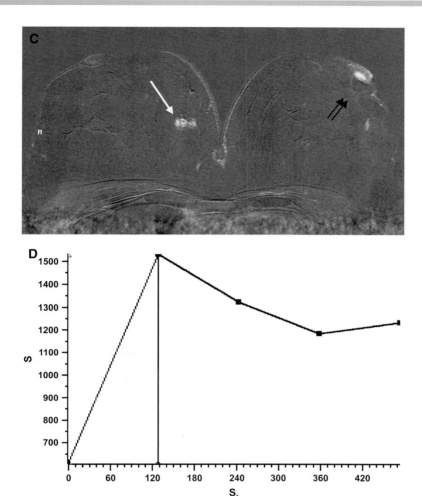

Fig. 5 (continued).

medullar invasive cancers. In MR imaging, differential diagnosis of medullar cancer versus fibroadenoma is possible because of the absence of dark internal septations, heterogeneous internal enhancement, or presence of a wash-out time course. The differential diagnosis of medullar cancer versus collapsed cysts is quite straightforward because of the absence of enhancement in collapsed cysts. Because of its ability to diagnose medullar cancer more reliably, MR imaging has an established role in the surveillance of women at high familial risk for breast cancer.

Lobular-invasive cancer (see Fig. 8) makes up approximately 10% to 15% of invasive breast cancers. Because of their "indian file" growth pattern, the tumors gradually replace the preexisting fibroglandular tissue. This peculiar growth pattern, together with the frequent lack of associated microcalcifications, seems to account for the fact that lobular-invasive breast cancer can go undetected by

mammography (and breast ultrasound) for a long time. On breast MR imaging, most lobular-invasive breast cancer appears as irregular masses. In approximately 20% of cases, an actual mass is missing; instead, the diffuse cellular infiltration of the parenchyma appears as asymmetric non–mass-like enhancement. It has been shown that in diffusely infiltrating lobular cancer, the entire process of angiogenesis is regulated by a different set of local tissue hormones compared with those released by invasive ductal cancers, for example. This is also intuitively plausible, because diffusely infiltrating single tumor cells can be nourished by diffusion through the existing capillaries of the fibroglandular tissue and do not need new vasculature for extra nutrient support. As a result, enhancement in diffusely infiltrating lobular cancer may be only slow and shallow, and no wash-out phenomenon should be expected. What follows is that if lobular-invasive breast cancer is a consideration, slow

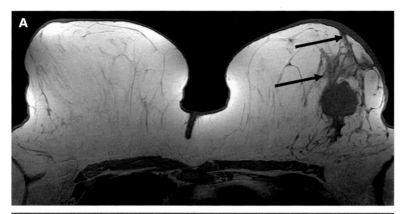

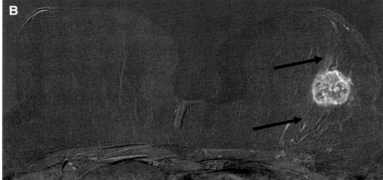

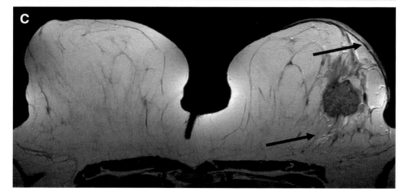

Fig. 6. Ductal invasive cancer with pronounced lymphangiosis in a 39-year-old patient. (*A*) Precontrast, T1-weighted, gradient echo image. (*B*) Postcontrast subtracted image. (*C*) T2-weighted non–fat-suppressed image. Note the round mass with relatively smooth borders, which may appear as a benign mass. Note, however, the pronounced rim enhancement, which is typical of invasive cancer. Note the thickened septa and the hazy enhancement around the cancer (*arrows*). This is peritumoral lymphangiosis. Note also the regional edema (*C*) and the skin thickening (*A, C*).

or shallow enhancement is not atypical but consistent with this diagnosis. The main differential diagnosis of diffusely infiltrating lobular cancer is chronic subclinical mastitis or, in case it happens to exhibit a segmental growth pattern, intraductal cancer (DCIS). It should be noted that in our experience, lobular-invasive breast cancer is overrepresented in women undergoing breast MR imaging, such that it made up 27% of all invasive cancers in our series.

Mucinous invasive cancer (Fig. 9) is usually well differentiated and occurs in elderly women. It accounts for approximately 2% to 5% of all breast cancers. A key feature of this cancer is a mass with irregular shape and borders and, depending on the degree of mucin production, an intermediate to high signal intensity in non–fat-suppressed T2-weighted images equivalent to fatty tissue or water-filled cysts. The more mucin is accumulated, the higher is the signal intensity in T2-weighted TSE images and the lower is the enhancement that occurs after contrast injection. Mucinous cancer accounts for most noninvasive or slowly enhancing invasive breast cancers published in case reports on invasive breast cancers missed by MR imaging. If they are entirely filled up with mucin, these cancers may best be identified on precontrast non–fat-suppressed

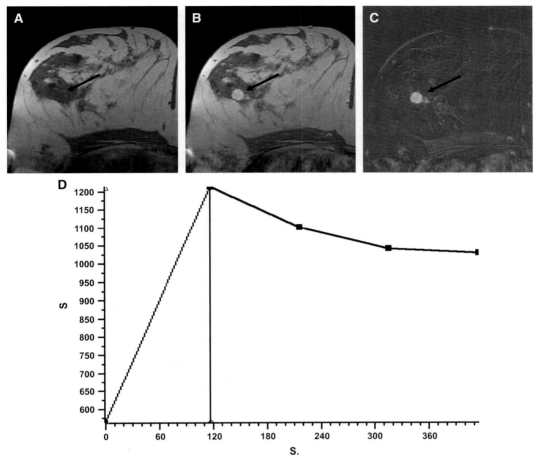

Fig. 7. Well-circumscribed breast cancer; value of additional kinetic analysis. Ductal invasive cancer in a 48-year-old patient. (*A*) Precontrast, T1-weighted, gradient echo image. (*B*) Early postcontrast image. (*C*) Postcontrast subtracted image. (*D*) Time/signal intensity curve of the enhancing mass. Note the round mass (*arrows*) with smooth borders and relatively homogeneous internal architecture. Note, however, the rapid early enhancement followed by a wash-out time course, which is typical for invasive cancer.

T1-weighted and T2-weighted images. Key to the diagnosis is a mass that exhibits signal intensity characteristics similar to a simple cyst, but unlike cysts, does show at least some faint central enhancement and, notably, is irregular and has a hyperechoic correlate on breast ultrasound. This combination (a seemingly cystic lesion with an irregular shape and [even faint] enhancement and bright echo at ultrasound) should always raise the suspicion of mucinous cancer.

Tubular invasive cancers are usually easy to diagnose because they present as stellate masses with spiculated borders, and a typical fast and strong enhancement, followed by wash-out. The main differential diagnosis is radial scars, and there are currently no definite criteria available that would reliably help to distinguish tubular cancer from (surrounding) radial scars.

Inflammatory breast cancer is a clinical rather than radiologic diagnosis. It presents clinically as an acute inflammation of a breast, with skin reddening, edema, and tenderness. It is categorized as pT4d (ie, the most advanced local tumor stage of the tumor node metastasis [TNM] classification system). Inflammatory breast cancer is caused by isolated breast cancer cells that diffusely infiltrate the fibroglandular tissue, with tumor cells spreading in the lymphatic channels. The obstruction of the lymphatic channels by infiltrating tumor cells causes the intramammary edema (see Fig. 6) and the inflammatory appearance. In mammography, there is diffusely increased density of the entire parenchyma, combined with skin thickening. The underlying cancer is often not seen, which makes the differential diagnosis of inflammatory cancer and acute mastitis difficult. The same holds true,

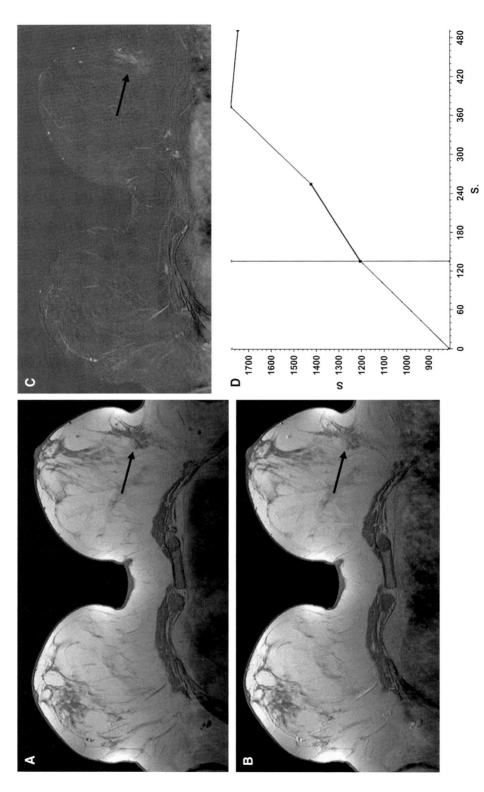

Fig. 8. Lobular invasive cancer in a 53-year-old patient. (A) Precontrast, T1-weighted, gradient echo image. (B) Early postcontrast subtracted image. (C) Early postcontrast image. (D) Time/signal intensity curve of the enhancing area, which exhibits persistent enhancement. Note there is non–mass-like enhancement that is asymmetric in the left upper outer quadrant. This is diffusely infiltrating lobular invasive cancer (*arrows*) with only shallow angiogenic activity and slow enhancement. In non–mass-like enhancement, a benign signal intensity time course with persistent enhancement cannot be used to alleviate the indication to perform a biopsy.

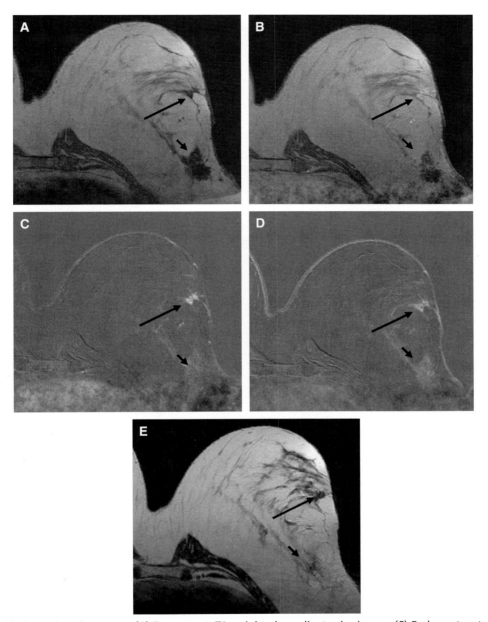

Fig. 9. Mucinous invasive cancer. (*A*) Precontrast, T1-weighted, gradient echo image. (*B*) Early postcontrast image. (*C*) Early postcontrast subtracted image. (*D*) Late postcontrast subtracted image. (*E*) T2-weighted non–fat-suppressed image. Note there are two masses: one in the retroareolar region in the anterior portion of the breast, (*long arrow*) and one in the posterior prepectoral portion (*short arrow*). Note the anterior mass exhibits typical cancer-like enhancement and signal intensity patterns. Note the posterior mass (*short arrow*) exhibits only faint and slow enhancement, which is visible only in the late postcontrast phase (*D*). Note that this mass exhibits very bright signal on a T2-weighted TSE image (*E*), which makes it isointense to fatty tissue. This is multifocal mucinous invasive cancer. One tumor (the one in the anterior location) consists of solid cancer and contains only little mucin; the second tumor has only scarce solid components and consists mainly of mucin.

however, for MR imaging. Here, diffuse enhancement of the entire fibroglandular tissue, often including the skin, is observed. Compared with the regular invasive breast cancer, inflammatory cancer may go along with only slow or subtle enhancement and may even not exhibit enhancement at all. Accordingly, breast MR imaging is not always helpful to distinguish inflammatory breast cancer and mastitis. If no enhancing mass is seen, the patient may still have inflammatory cancer.

Intraductal cancers (ductal carcinoma in situ)

DCIS (Fig. 10) exhibits a variable degree of angiogenic activity, and thus enhancement in breast MR imaging. Because, by definition, DCIS is a lesion that is confined to the intraductal epithelium, it is surprising that DCIS does, in fact, enhance in breast MR imaging at all, because this suggests that these lesions do, in fact, interact with the periductal stroma to initiate periductal angiogenesis. In general, the wash-in rate (early rise) of contrast agent in DCIS is lower compared with what is observed in invasive breast cancers. Unlike the situation in invasive breast cancers, absence of enhancement is

observed in 5% to 10% of cases of DCIS. Because of the lack of enhancement, these cases of DCIS are not detectable by breast MR imaging. This is one of the major reasons why a mammogram is still considered a necessary prerequisite for the interpretation of a breast MR imaging study. This is the reason why breast MR imaging cannot be used to alleviate the indication to perform a biopsy of mammographic findings that are suspicious for DCIS. Conversely, approximately 20% of cases of DCIS that do exhibit enhancement and are therefore diagnosed by breast MR imaging do not exhibit calcifications on a mammogram, such that lack of

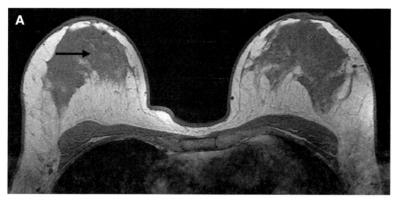

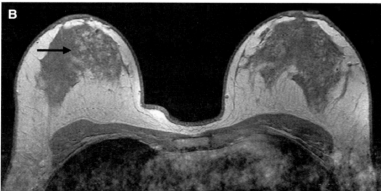

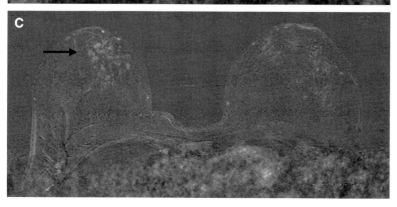

Fig. 10. Intraductal cancer in a 48-year-old patient. (*A*) Precontrast, T1-weighted, gradient echo image. (*B*) Postcontrast image. (*C*) Postcontrast subtracted image. Note the non–mass-like enhancement in a segmental distribution (*arrow*). Note the clumped internal enhancement. Note that the enhancement is slow and shallow compared with the enhancement in invasive cancers like those in Fig. 1 or 4. Typical appearance of DCIS.

calcifications in a mammogram cannot be used to alleviate the indication to perform a biopsy an enhancing area that is suggestive of DCIS in breast MR imaging.

Approximately half of the cases of enhancing DCIS exhibit rather shallow enhancement; in these cases, the time course is virtually always persistent (ie, benign). The other half of cases of DCIS reveal early enhancement; however, even then, a wash-out time course is rare. Accordingly, kinetic features cannot be used to diagnose DCIS or, more precisely, absence of cancer-type fast enhancement, and wash-out may not be used to alleviate the indication to perform a biopsy of an enhancing area that is suspicious for DCIS. Accordingly the diagnosis is mainly based on the assessment of lesion morphology (eg, configuration, distribution). Most cases of DCIS do not appear as masses. Instead, non–mass-like enhancement that follows the ductal system is the hallmark of DCIS in breast MR imaging. Non–mass-like enhancement with asymmetric (ie, unilateral) ductal or segmental distribution is attributable to DCIS in at least 30% of cases; in other words, this finding has a high positive predictive value (PPV) for intraductal cancer. Because breast MR imaging is able to demonstrate DCIS that does not exhibit calcifications on mammography, ductal or segmental enhancement should entail a biopsy. Less often (in approximately 20% of cases), DCIS may appear as a focus, focal area, or regional enhancement. Intraductal tumor that spreads within and around an invasive cancer is referred to as an extensive intraductal component (EIC) and is considered one of the few remaining contraindications for breast-conserving surgery. In breast MR imaging, an EIC appears as non–mass-like enhancement that extends from an invasive cancer, usually with less pronounced enhancement than the invasive component.

If an intraductal cancer is sufficiently large, internal enhancement can be evaluated. It is almost always heterogeneous, exhibiting an enhancement pattern that has been referred to as being granular, stippled, or clumped.

Although there are reports stating that high-resolution breast MR imaging is able to visualize DCIS-induced microcalcifications, most researchers cannot confirm this. In practice, and with currently available hardware, it still holds true that breast MR imaging does not allow visualization of microcalcifications. Hence, analysis of microcalcifications cannot be exploited to detect or classify DCIS in breast MR imaging.

Lobular carcinoma in situ

This lesion is still considered to represent a marker lesion of increased breast cancer risk rather than a direct precursor of breast cancer that would require therapy to avoid invasive breast cancer (as is the case in DCIS). Still, diagnosis of lobular carcinoma in situ (LCIS) does have an impact on patient management in that the patient is considered to carry an increased risk for breast cancer and may require intensified surveillance. In fact, in a recent study, women who were diagnosed with LCIS had a substantially increased risk of subsequent invasive breast cancer, more often of the ductal type than of the lobular type, yet with more lobular cancers than in the average population. The risk is increased for the ipsilateral breast and, albeit to a lower extent, for the opposite breast. Pleomorphic LCIS is a subgroup of LCIS that has been shown to go along with an increased risk of subsequent lobular invasive cancers and is meanwhile considered to be a true precursor (rather than only a marker) lesion. In breast MR imaging, as in mammography, there is no finding that is specific for LCIS in that it would allow the prospective diagnosis of LCIS. In our experience, LCIS may appear just as mastopathic changes, focal adenosis, or DCIS.

Breast MR imaging features of benign tumors: fibroadenomas

As has long been established by conventional breast imaging modalities (mammography and high-frequency breast ultrasound), morphologic features are of utmost importance for the correct classification of benign lesions. Fibroadenomas (Figs. 11 and 12) appear as masses, almost always with a roundish, oval, or lobular shape and with smooth margins. All further MR imaging features of fibroadenomas vary with their histologic subtype (see Fig. 11). The so-called juvenile or myxoid fibroadenomas contain a gelatinous interstitial matrix that undergoes progressive fibrosis and gradually result in so-called "sclerotic" (fibrotic) fibroadenomas. Myxoid fibroadenomas exhibit fast enhancement with a persistent time course. Usually, enhancement starts in the center of the mass and progresses from there to the lesion periphery. Because of this centrifugal progression of enhancement, fibroadenomas may look misleadingly irregular in the early postcontrast phase when enhancement of the tumors is still incomplete. The same holds true when partial fibrosis has occurred and only part of the fibroadenoma (the nonsclerotic part) exhibits enhancement. Diagnostic errors can be avoided by including precontrast, nonsubtracted, non–fat-suppressed images into the image analysis. On non–fat-suppressed T2-weighted images, myxoid fibroadenomas exhibit a high signal intensity compared with the adjacent fibroglandular tissue (yet usually not as high as fatty tissue or cysts).

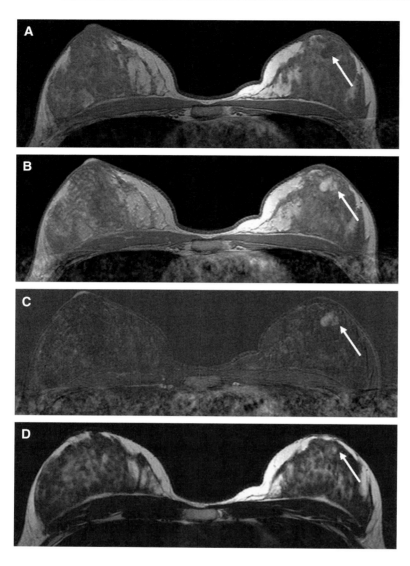

Fig. 11. Myxoid fibroadenoma. (*A*) Precontrast, T1-weighted, gradient echo image. (*B*) Early postcontrast image. (*C*) Early postcontrast subtracted image. (*D*) T2-weighted non–fat-suppressed image. Note the lobular enhancing mass with smooth borders (*arrows*). Note that internal septations are visible. Note the relatively high signal in the T2-weighted TSE image compared with the adjacent fibroglandular tissue. Typical fibroadenoma.

This is in contrast to most invasive breast cancers, which tend to exhibit low signal intensity (isointense to fibroglandular tissue) on T2-weighted TSE images. Internal enhancement of myxoid fibroadenomas is homogeneous, or dark internal septations are visible. The latter are only visible in pulse sequences that use a high spatial resolution. Dark internal septations offer a high negative predictive value for breast cancer. In our department, if an oval mass with smooth borders exhibits internal septations, the lesion is categorized as definitely benign.

Sclerotic fibroadenomas (see Fig. 12) exhibit only weak enhancement or no enhancement at all. Therefore, they may be missed if only subtracted or fat-suppressed postcontrast images are evaluated. Internal architecture is usually not evaluable because of the absence of enhancement. Dark internal

septations are usually not perceivable, because the entire lesion is isointense to the signal of the septa in all pulse sequences. Sclerotic fibroadenomas are best visualized on non–fat-suppressed, TSE, T2-weighted images, where they appear as a roundish mass with smooth borders and exhibit an extremely hypointense signal darker than that of the pectoral muscle.

Nodular mastopathic changes and focal adenosis

So-called "nodular-mastopathic" changes and focal adenosis are notorious causes of diagnostic difficulties (see Fig. 3; Fig. 13). When one starts reading breast MR imaging studies, one is surprised at how many tiny roundish foci of enhancement can be seen. It is virtually impossible to try and classify each and every enhancing spot in these cases. If, for

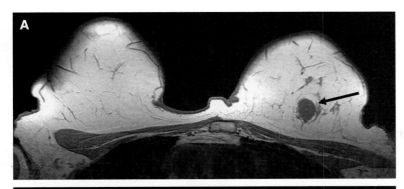

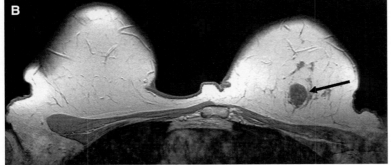

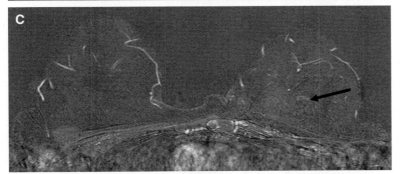

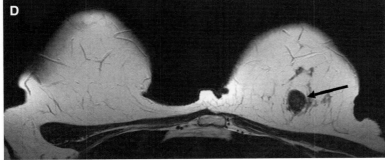

Fig. 12. Sclerotic fibroadenoma in a 48-year-old patient with a suspicious ultrasound finding in the left breast in the 12 o'clock position. (*A*) Precontrast, T1-weighted, gradient echo image. (*B*) Early postcontrast image. (*C*) Early postcontrast subtracted image. (*D*) T2-weighted non–fat-suppressed image. Note that the lesion is invisible on the postcontrast subtracted image (*C*) because of the absence of enhancement. Note the round mass (*arrows*) with smooth margins in the pre- and postcontrast nonsubtracted images (*A, B*) and the low signal intensity of the lesion in the T2-weighted, TSE, non–fat-suppressed image (*D*). The findings are typical for sclerotic fibroadenoma.

one reason or another, one of these foci happens to be biopsied, the histologic report usually mentions small foci of adenosis/epitheliosis, small fibroadenomas, solitary small papillomas, a mixture of all that, or no findings at all but just plain breast parenchyma. The actual problem with these lesions is that they are too small and too numerous to allow

a clear-cut differential diagnosis: most (if not all) differential criteria mentioned do not work in extremely small (≤5 mm) lesions because of insufficient spatial resolution or partial volume averaging as well as biologic issues. Kinetic features are not necessarily helpful either, because many of these foci exhibit fast, strong, early enhancement and

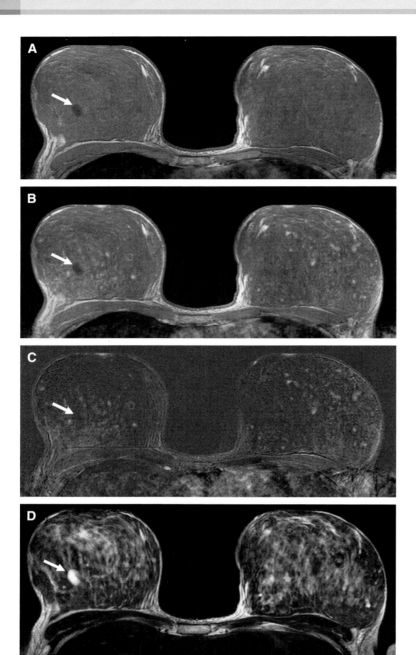

Fig. 13. Focal adenosis in a 52-year-old patient. (*A*) Precontrast, T1-weighted, gradient echo image. (*B*) Early postcontrast image. (*C*) Early postcontrast subtracted image. (*D*) Non-fat suppressed T2-weighted image. Note the multiple foci of enhancement that are disseminated in both breasts. Note that the foci are more or less symmetric on both sides and do not follow the distribution of the milk ducts. Note a cyst in the right breast with low signal on the T1-weighted image pre- and post-contrast, no enhancement, and bright signal on T2-weighted TSE images (*short white arrow*).

even a wash-out time course. Thus, the question is one of how these lesions should be managed.

In general, management depends on the clinical and medicolegal setting. If these foci are identified in a patient who has a history of breast cancer or carries an increased risk for breast cancer, follow-up is usually the best decision. Focal adenosis is usually relatively stable, however, and does not resolve on follow-up. Because lack of growth is a relatively weak criterion to exclude breast cancer, it takes several follow-up studies to settle the

problem. If a patient has no increased risk of breast cancer and multiple foci are identified in both breasts, we code them as BI-RADS 2 and leave them alone, provided, of course, that there is no clinical, mammographic, or ultrasound correlate for the enhancing foci.

Hormonal stimulation

One of the most important causes for non–mass-like enhancement in breast MR imaging is endogenous as well as exogenous hormones. There is evidence that ovarian hormones exhibit a hista-mine-like effect on the fibroglandular tissue that seems to induce regional or focal hyperemia, which is why normal breast parenchyma may be found at histologic examination if these lesions undergo biopsy. It has been extensively documented that these lesions are particularly prevalent in young premenopausal patients, that they arise and disappear along with the menstrual cycle, and that they may recur if hormonal replacement therapy (HRT) is initiated in postmenopausal patients. Hormone-induced enhancement appears as non–mass-like enhancement, usually not following the ductal system but as foci, solitary or multiple focal areas or as regional or diffuse enhancement. Although in most cases, slowly progressive enhancement is seen, depending on the degree of hormonal stimulation, rapid enhancement may be observed in up to 40% of cases. Even if rapid enhancement occurs, however, it is usually persistent, whereas a wash-out time course is extremely rare. Although this sounds reassuring, it is not extremely helpful, because wash-out is rarely seen in any non–mass-like enhancing lesion, including malignant lesions (eg, DCIS, lobular cancer). In view of the serious diagnostic difficulties that may be caused by hormonal stimulation, it seems wise to try to avoid hormonal stimulation whenever possible or to exploit its transient nature. In young premenopausal patients, the lowest prevalence of hormonal-induced enhancement was found in the second week of the menstrual cycle. Elective breast MR imaging studies in young premenopausal women (eg, undergoing screening for familial cancer) should be scheduled for this week if at all possible. If findings consistent with hormonal stimulation are still encountered, follow-up after one or two menstrual periods is the best way to deal with them. In postmenopausal patients on HRT, discontinuing medication for 6 weeks has been shown to be sufficient to reduce the prevalence of hormone-induced enhancement.

Cysts

Regular cysts appear as smoothly bordered round-ish or oval masses without any enhancement and bright signal on fat-suppressed or non–fat-suppressed, TSE, T2-weighted images (see Fig. 13, long arrow). With increasing proteinaceous content of the cysts, signal on TSE T2-weighted images decreases and that on precontrast T1-weighted images increases (see Fig. 3, thick arrow). Because of the complete absence of enhancement even in the late postcontrast phase, however, there are no difficulties in differential diagnosis. Accordingly, breast MR imaging is well suited to help distinguish collapsed or proteinaceous cysts (which may appear

suspicious on breast ultrasound) from well-defined breast cancer. This is especially useful in high-risk women with familiar breast cancer, who are known to exhibit benign morphologic features frequently. In complicated cysts, enhancement may occur in the tissue around the cyst (Fig. 14). Again, this may appear as mass with rim enhancement on subtracted images. Reference to non–fat-suppressed nonsubtracted images should help to avoid diagnostic errors.

Postsurgical scar

After major breast surgery, fresh scars may exhibit contrast enhancement. It is difficult to predict at which time interval after surgery no enhancement occurs; usually, the interval is set to 6 months. In individual cases, however, this may vary considerably; in women with complicated wound healing, enhancement may persist for a longer period, and other women do not have any enhancement at all only a few weeks after surgery. In any case, enhancement of scars should not provoke serious differential diagnostic problems. This is because scar enhancement is relatively subtle and occurs more or less evenly in the entire scar. This is in contrast to recurrent cancer, which exhibits a mass effect within the scar and causes focal enhancement that is confined to a part of the scar. Accordingly, even in the early postcontrast phase, breast MR imaging can be safely performed to distinguish scar from recurrent or residual breast cancer. The situation may be more difficult in cases in which fat necrosis develops in the scar or close to it, because fatty tissue necrosis may cause focal, early, and strong enhancement within a scar.

Fat necrosis

Postoperative fat necrosis (oil cysts) (see Fig. 5 double arrow) is usually easy to diagnose. It appears as a mass with central fatty tissue and a fibrous capsule (ie, lesion with a dark [low signal intensity] rim and bright signal in the center on nonsubtracted and non–fat-suppressed T1- and T2-weighted images). In acute fat necrosis, there is an inflammatory reaction in the fibrous capsule, which goes along with enhancement of the dark rim. Accordingly, in fat-suppressed or subtracted images, this may appear as a mass with rim enhancement and could be mixed up with an enhancing invasive cancer. If non–fat-suppressed and nonsubtracted images are evaluated, however, the central fatty tissue becomes obvious, which facilitates the diagnosis. If no central fatty tissue is observed, it is impossible to distinguish recurrent cancer from fatty tissue necrosis. In our department, if fat necrosis is a differential diagnostic consideration, we schedule the patient for

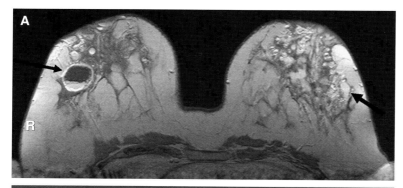

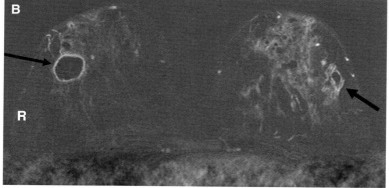

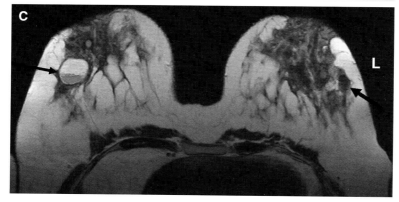

Fig. 14. Bilateral complicated cysts and duct ectasia in a 52-year-old patient. (*A*) Precontrast, T1-weighted, gradient echo image. (*B*) Early postcontrast image. (*C*) T2-weighted TSE image. Note the masses in both breasts with rim enhancement. Note that the enhancing rim occurs around the two masses (cysts) rather than within the mass. Note that cyst on the right (*long arrows*) shows acute hemorrhage (typical bright signal on precontrast T1-weighted images and intermediate signal on T2-weighted TSE images) with a fluid/fluid level; the one on the left (*short arrows*) exhibits high precontrast on T1-weighted images and low signal on T2-weighted TSE images because of proteinaceous content.

short-term follow-up, because the inflammatory reaction that causes the enhancement in fresh fat necrosis is usually rapidly reversible. If the expected change of enhancement is not observed on follow-up and the picture is unchanged, we recommend biopsy.

Radial scar (complex sclerosing lesion)

Just as in mammography, a radial scar presents as a stellate lesion, usually without mass effect. Unfortunately, not only morphology but enhancement kinetics of radial scars may mimic those of invasive breast cancers. Therefore, a clear-cut distinction of a radial scar versus invasive cancer is usually not possible; accordingly, breast MR imaging cannot

be used to help distinguish a radial scar from breast cancer or to help identify tubular cancer in the periphery of a radial scar.

Intramammary lymph nodes

Intramammary lymph nodes are a frequent finding. Most often, they are located in the subcutaneous fatty tissue or embedded in the superficial part of the fibroglandular tissue of the upper outer quadrant. In subtracted or fat-suppressed MR imaging, normal lymph nodes appear as roundish or oval masses with smooth borders and strong and fast enhancement, followed by wash-out. Accordingly, they may be mixed up with cancer. This is particularly true in lymph nodes with a prominent central hilum that contains fatty tissue, and thus does not enhance after contrast agent injection. This results in a mass with rim enhancement (ie, enhancing lymphatic ring around a nonenhancing fatty tissue hilum). Again, reference to the non–fat-suppressed or nonsubtracted images should help to clarify the situation. As opposed to breast cancer, intramammary lymph nodes exhibit an oval, round, or (ideally) kidney shape with smooth borders. Unlike breast cancer, there is a central fatty tissue signal that clinches the diagnosis. Enhancement kinetics are always suspicious (ie, exhibit fast and strong enhancement with wash-out) even in normal lymph nodes. Accordingly, enhancement kinetics are misleading and cannot be used to distinguish intramammary lymph nodes from breast cancer or to distinguish normal from diseased (or metastatic) intramammary lymph nodes.

Mastitis

In acute mastitis, all typical clinical signs of inflammation are usually present, with breast swelling, tenderness, and skin reddening. Systemic symptoms, such as fever, elevated white blood cell count, and elevated C-reactive protein (CRP), are less consistently found. In MR imaging, there is extensive edema of the fibroglandular tissue and the skin, which is best visualized on fat-suppressed or non–fat-suppressed, TSE, T2-weighted images. Usually, the entire fibroglandular tissue and the skin exhibit diffuse enhancement. If abscess formation occurs, there are masses with rapid and strong rim enhancement. Differentiation from breast cancer is usually feasible, because pus formation is associated with high signal intensity on precontrast T1-weighted images. The main differential diagnosis

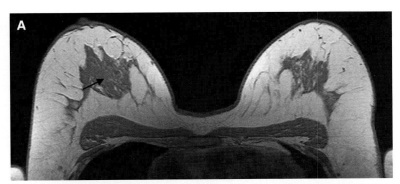

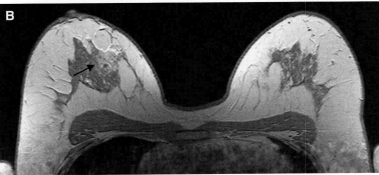

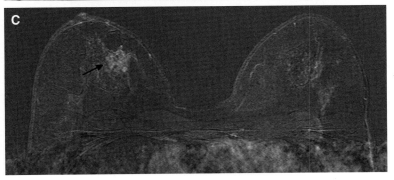

Fig. 15. Chronic mastitis in a 49-year-old patient. (*A*) Precontrast, T1-weighted, gradient echo image. (*B*) Early postcontrast image. (*C*) Early postcontrast subtracted image. Note the non–mass-like enhancement (*arrows*). The main differential diagnosis is DCIS or lobular-invasive cancer.

of diffusely enhancing acute mastitis is inflammatory breast cancer. Currently, there are no diagnostic criteria available that would allow a clear-cut differentiation between these two entities.

In chronic mastitis (Fig. 15), clinical signs and symptoms of inflammation may be entirely lacking, which makes the diagnosis even more difficult. Chronic mastitis may go along with regional or focal non–mass-related or mass-related enhancement. As such, it is usually indistinguishable from DCIS or diffusely infiltrating lobular invasive cancer.

In chronic granulomatous mastitis, rim-enhancing masses may be observed. As opposed to rim-enhancing cancers, these lesions tend to exhibit central high signal intensity in TSE T2-weighted images; they appear relatively well circumscribed and are usually clustered. A cluster of multiple aggregated rim-enhancing masses is relatively rarely caused by breast cancer. Accordingly, although the diagnosis can be suspected by breast MR imaging, a biopsy is still required to facilitate safe differentiation from breast cancer.

Suggested readings

American College of Radiology (ACR). ACR BI-RADSR–magnetic resonance imaging. In: ACR breast imaging reporting and data system, breast imaging atlas. Reston (VA): American College of Radiology; 2003.

Hochman MG, Orel SG, Powell CM, et al. Fibroadenomas: MR imaging appearances with radiologic-histopathologic correlation. Radiology 1997;204:123–9.

Ikeda O, Nishimura R, Miyayama H, et al. Magnetic resonance evaluation of the presence of an extensive intraductal component in breast cancer. Acta Radiol 2004;45:721–5.

Kinkel K, Helbich TH, Esserman LJ, et al. Dynamic high-spatial-resolution MR imaging of suspicious breast lesions: diagnostic criteria and interobserver variability. AJR Am J Roentgenol 2000;175:35–43.

Kuhl CK, Bieling HB, Gieseke J, et al. Healthy premenopausal breast parenchyma in dynamic contrast-enhanced MR imaging of the breast: normal contrast medium enhancement and cyclical-phase dependency. Radiology 1997;203:137–44.

Kuhl CK, Mielcarek P, Klaschik S, et al. Are signal time course data useful for differential diagnosis of enhancing lesions in dynamic breast MR imaging? Radiology 1999;211:101–10.

Kuhl CK, Mielcarek P, Klaschik S, et al. Are T2-weighted pulse sequences helpful to assist differential diagnosis of enhancing lesions in dynamic breast MRI? J Magn Reson Imaging 1999;9:187–96.

Liberman L, Morris EA, Dershaw DD, et al. Ductal enhancement on MR imaging of the breast. AJR Am J Roentgenol 2003;181:519–25.

Morakkabati-Spitz N, Leutner C, Schild HH, et al. Diagnostic usefulness of segmental and linear enhancement in dynamic breast MRI. Eur Radiol 2005;15:2010–7.

Müller-Schimpfle M, Ohmenhauser K, Stoll P, et al. Menstrual cycle and age: influence on parenchymal contrast medium enhancement in MR imaging of the breast. Radiology 1997;203:145–9.

Nunes LW, Schnall MD, Orel SG, et al. Breast MR imaging: interpretation model. Radiology 1997;202:833–41.

Nunes LW, Schnall MD, Siegelman ES, et al. Diagnostic performance characteristics of architectural features revealed by high spatial-resolution MR imaging of the breast. AJR Am J Roentgenol 1997;169:409–15.

Orel SG. High-resolution MR imaging of the breast. Semin Ultrasound CT MR 1996;17:476–93.

Qayyum A, Birdwell RL, Daniel BL, et al. MR imaging features of infiltrating lobular carcinoma of the breast: histopathologic correlation. AJR Am J Roentgenol 2002;178:1227–32.

Yeh ED, Slanetz PJ, Edmister WB, et al. Invasive lobular carcinoma: spectrum of enhancement and morphology on magnetic resonance imaging. Breast J 2003;9:13–8.

References

[1] Folkman J, Klagsbrun M. Angiogenic factors. Science 1987;235:442–7.

[2] Folkman J, Watson K, Ingbr D, et al. Induction of angiogenesis during the transition from hyperplasia to neoplasia. Nature 1989;339:58–61.

[3] Kaiser WA, Zeitler E. MR imaging of the breast: fast imaging sequences with and without Gd-DTPA. Preliminary observations. Radiology 1989;170:681–6.

[4] Heywang SH, Wolf A, Pruss E, et al. MR imaging of the breast with Gd-DTPA: use and limitations. Radiology 1989;171:95–103.

[5] Harms SE, Flamig DP, Hesley KL, et al. MR imaging of the breast with rotating delivery of excitation off resonance: clinical experience with pathologic correlation. Radiology 1993;187:493–501.

[6] Kuhl CK, Schild HH, Morakkabati N. On the trade-off between spatial and temporal resolution in dynamic bilateral contrast enhanced MRI of the breast. Radiology 2005;236:789–800.

[7] Perlet C, Heinig A, Prat X, et al. Multicenter study for the evaluation of a dedicated biopsy device for MR-guided vacuum biopsy of the breast. Eur Radiol 2002;12:1463–70.

[8] Kuhl CK, Elevelt A, Leutner C, et al. Clinical use of a stereotactic localization and biopsy device for interventional breast MRI. Radiology 1997;204(3):667–75.

[9] Liberman L, Bracero N, Morris E, et al. MRI-guided 9-gauge vacuum-assisted breast biopsy: initial clinical experience. AJR Am J Roentgenol 2005;185:183–93.

[10] Ikeda DM, Hylton NM, Kinkel K, et al. Development, standardization, and testing of a lexicon for reporting contrast-enhanced breast magnetic resonance imaging studies. J Magn Reson Imaging 2001;13:889–95.

ELSEVIER
SAUNDERS

MAGNETIC
RESONANCE
IMAGING CLINICS

Magn Reson Imaging Clin N Am 14 (2006) 329–337

Breast MR Imaging in the Diagnostic Setting

Mitchell Schnall, MD, PhD*, Susan Orel, MD

- MR imaging diagnosis of primary breast cancer
- Multicenter results from the International Breast MR Imaging Consortium
- Practical implementation of MR imaging in the diagnostic setting
- Summary
- References

Breast cancer screening with mammography has been shown to reduce breast cancer–specific mortality in several randomized studies [1–3], and at present, mammography remains the primary imaging modality used to detect early clinically occult breast cancer. Despite advances in mammographic technique, however, limitations remain. One major limitation of mammography is overlap in appearances of benign and malignant lesions. Because of this, lesions are assigned a Breast Imaging and Reporting Data System (BI-RADS) assessment of 4 if they are thought to be in the range of 2% to 90% likely to be malignant. Thus, lesions over a wide range of suspicion are placed in a category of being recommended for biopsy. The overlap in the mammographic appearance and physical examination findings of benign and malignant lesions results in a relatively high number of benign breast biopsies. The resultant positive predictive value for mammography is approximately 15% to 30% [4]. Given the implication of missed cancer on the care of a woman and the current medical legal climate in the United States, breast imagers tend to operate in the high-sensitivity part of the receiver operating characteristic (ROC) curve, and thus choose to perform a biopsy rather than follow lesions even with a small likelihood of being malignant. Although the high number of benign excisional biopsies has been greatly reduced with the implementation of percutaneous needle core biopsy [5], the problem of false-positive mammographic findings results in unnecessary patient anxiety and morbidity related to the biopsy as well as to increased health care costs.

The high benign biopsy rate has generated significant interest in adjunctive imaging tests that would improve the positive predictive value of the diagnostic workup of findings in the breast detected during screening. To have clinical value, the adjunctive modality must have an extremely high negative predictive value—high enough to downgrade lesions from "suspicious" to "probably benign" or "benign." Thus, in this role, it is the ability to classify a finding as definitively benign that is required rather than the ability to detect cancer. The classic example of an adjunctive modality that has been successfully used to improve specificity of screening is sonography [6]. Women with one or more masses on mammography are often evaluated with sonography to determine if the mass or masses represent cysts. Simple cysts are usually diagnosed definitively with sonography. These simple cysts are benign and placed into BI-RADS category 2 and are assumed to be benign. The use of directed ultrasound serves as

Department of Radiology, Hospital of the University of Pennsylvania, 3400 Spruce Street, Philadelphia, PA 19104, USA
* Corresponding author.
E-mail address: schnall@oasis.rad.upenn.edu (M. Schnall).

doi:10.1016/j.mric.2006.07.004

a potential model for the use of any adjunctive breast imaging test.

Among adjunctive approaches currently being proposed for improving sensitivity are MR imaging, ^{18}F-fluorodeoxyglucose (FDG) positron emission tomography [7], [99]Tc- sestamibi scintigraphy [8], and expanding the use of sonography [6]. Although still under investigation, the nuclear medicine techniques have not received large-scale acceptance because of limitations in imaging smaller lesions and concerns that some tumors have physiology such that they are not avid for FDG, leading to false-negative findings. The use of sonography to characterize solid lesions better as proposed by Stavoros and colleagues [6] is gaining more widespread use, in part, because of the long-standing experience with sonography in the diagnostic setting and availability of sonography in most breast imaging centers. Thus, in some centers, not all solid masses that undergo sonographic evaluation are assessed as suspicious requiring biopsy. Solid lesions displaying benign characteristics are assessed as 2 (benign) or 3 (probably benign).

MR imaging has been proposed as a technique with a high negative predictive value and, as such, is gaining more widespread use in the diagnostic setting. In the diagnostic setting, the role of breast MR imaging is that of an adjunct to conventional imaging (mammography and/or sonography) and clinical examination to characterize appropriate equivocal findings further.

MR imaging diagnosis of primary breast cancer

Although the results of early clinical investigation of MR imaging of the breast suggested that the presence of signal enhancement after contrast injection would be a sensitive and specific sign for malignancy [9], it became clear that enhancement alone was not specific for cancer [10,11]. Harms and colleagues [11] performed careful correlation between breast MR imaging and mastectomy specimens in a population of women undergoing mastectomy for breast cancer. They observed an overall sensitivity of 94% for the visualization of breast cancer, detecting occult cancer by mammography in 37% of women. This speaks to the high sensitivity of MR imaging. They observed that only approximately 40% of the enhancing foci detected by MR imaging were cancer, however [11].

Over past decade, there has been extensive clinical investigation into developing strategies to reduce false-positive MR imaging findings. Proposed strategies include assessing the absolute maximum intensity of contrast enhancement, the kinetics of enhancement over time, lesion architectural features, or a combination of enhancement kinetics and architecture [10–17].

The initial technical approaches to breast MR imaging acquired images with relatively low spatial resolution, and thus were not ideal for evaluation of lesion architecture. Therefore, the initial approaches to the differential diagnosis in breast MR imaging were based on enhancement amplitude and kinetics. There has been extensive literature exploring the use of enhancement kinetics for the differential diagnosis of enhancing breast lesions [13–17]. Many of the approaches involved attempts to develop quantitative metrics for enhancement rates, amplitudes, or other parameters related to the enhancement kinetics. For example, Boetes and coworkers [13] placed a premium on high-time resolution. Their protocol consists of single-slice, non–fat-suppressed, gradient echo images with 2.6 mmol × 1.3 mmol in-plane spatial resolution (10-mmol slice) at 2.3-second time intervals. They used a criterion that any lesion with visible enhancement less than 11.5 seconds after arterial enhancement was considered suspicious for cancer. This criterion resulted in 95% sensitivity and 86% specificity for the diagnosis of cancer in a limited population. Citing problems in determining the proper location on the precontrast images to perform a single-slice dynamic examination and the need to detect other lesions within the breast, other investigators have recommended a multislice technique that records dynamic data from the entire breast after the injection of contrast [9]. These investigators have used multislice two-dimensional (2D) gradient echo, three-dimensional (3D) gradient echo, and echo planar techniques with time resolution varying from 12 seconds to 1 minute and widely distributed spatial resolution and section thickness. Criteria used to differentiate benign from malignant lesions have also varied widely among investigators. Criteria as simple as the percent enhancement at 2 minutes to more complex physiologic models that take into account the initial T1 of the lesion to estimate gadolinium (Gd) concentration as a function of time to extract pharmacokinetic parameters have been reported [14,15,18]. The accuracies cited by these investigators for interpretation based on contrast enhancement kinetics for differentiating benign from malignant lesions vary from 66% to 93%.

Although many investigators published near-perfect performance of their individual approach, this literature is characterized by small potentially biased patient samples. Furthermore, many of the quantitative techniques used were specific to a particular acquisition because of the strong dependence of quantitative enhancement on the scanning technique. These factors have limited the generalizability of these results. There is little use of quantitative kinetic analysis in routine clinical practice today. The most popular approach clinically has been the qualitative classification of enhancement curves at demonstrating persistent, plateau, or wash-out enhancement, however [17]. This approach has gained popularity because it is largely independent of imaging technique and technology. Versions of the qualitative approach have been adopted by vendors, resulting in products that allow qualitative and semiquantitative analysis to be used easily in a clinical setting.

Despite the many different techniques and results cited previously, it is clear that there is a tendency for cancer to enhance more rapidly than benign lesions after the bolus intravenous injection of Gd-chelate. It is also clear, however, that despite any technique and interpretation criterion used, there is some overlap in the dynamic curves between cancer and benign lesions. This has resulted in false-negative diagnoses in all series. The false-negative results are particularly problematic in considering the use of MR imaging in a diagnostic setting, where a high negative predictive value (close to 100%) is required. This is not surprising when one considers the variable histology of breast cancer. Cancer can form a solid tumor that is densely packed with epithelial tumor cells or can adopt a more infiltrative pattern with malignant ducts and epithelial cells intermixed with normal breast stroma (Fig. 1). In the latter case, typical MR imaging spatial resolution results in partial volume averaging between normal stroma and tumor elements. Thus, the contrast kinetics would be a weighted average of the various tissues included in the pixel. This contributes to the variable behavior of contrast kinetics across different cancers.

In addition to contrast kinetics, the architecture of enhancing lesions can be used to predict a diagnosis. Among the initial efforts to develop criteria for distinguishing benign from malignant breast lesions based on lesion architecture was the recursive partitioning interpretation scheme developed by Nunes and colleagues [12]. These investigators initially classified enhancement based on focal mass, ductal, or regional enhancement. Within each major category, classification was based on features specific to that category. For example, masses were classified by mass margin, T2 signal intensity, the presence of rim enhancement (associated with a high likelihood of malignancy), and the presence of nonenhancing internal septations (associated with a high likelihood of fibroadenoma). This scheme resulted in 95% sensitivity and 86% specificity for the diagnosis of cancer in a limited population. It also formed the basis for a preliminary version of a lexicon for breast MR imaging that had been initially developed by the Breast MR Imaging Working Group and continues to be supported and refined by a working group of the American College of Radiology [19].

Much of the controversy in the literature regarding the use of contrast enhancement kinetics as the primary interpretation criteria for breast MR imaging stems from the inherent trade-off that was required between spatial and temporal resolution. The technology available in the mid-1990s made it difficult to acquire images fast enough to follow the kinetics of enhancement with enough spatial resolution to observe the subtle architecture of enhancing lesions. More recently, technology has advanced, and combined approaches have been shown to offer the best results [15–17,20,21]. Today, most experts agree that breast MR imaging interpretation, with respect to classification of lesions as benign or malignant, should be based on morphologic appearance and contrast enhancement kinetics. A significant improvement in the

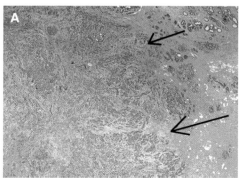 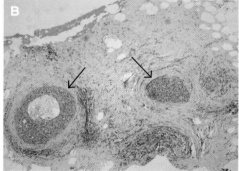

Fig. 1. (A) Hematoxylin-eosin (HE)–stained slide shows a dense cellular invasive tumor that demonstrates intensive enhancement on MR imaging. (B) HE-stained slide demonstrates foci of ductal carcinoma in situ (*arrows*) mixed with benign glands and stroma. Note that most of the tissue in the section is stroma. This lesion was occult to MR imaging.

diagnostic accuracy of breast MR imaging was demonstrated by Nunes and coworkers [16] after integrating kinetic data into the architectural model. In addition, Kuhl and coworkers [17,22] have advocated a combined approach to interpretation of breast MR imaging.

Multicenter results from the International Breast MR Imaging Consortium

The generalized diagnostic performance of breast MR imaging can be best assessed by the results of the multi-institutional trial conducted by the International Breast MR Imaging Consortium (IBMC). The IBMC study included 1004 women across 14 institutions with suspicious mammograms or clinical findings. This study found that the overall diagnostic performance of MR imaging as it is implemented and interpreted in most clinical centers was not sufficient to avoid biopsy in a cohort of all women presenting with an abnormal mammogram and/or physical examination without regard to the specifics of their presentation [23]. Although the IBMC study showed a higher positive predictive value for MR imaging compared with mammography in this setting (72.4% versus 52.8%), the sensitivity was not sufficient to exclude cancer reliably. The overall sensitivity in this population was reported to be 88%. The sensitivity for invasive cancer was 90.9%, whereas that for ductal carcinoma in situ (DCIS) was 73%. A significant finding was that the sensitivity for cancer in patients who presented with microcalcifications was lower than for those who presented with other findings (83.5 versus 90.3), although the overall accuracy of breast MR imaging was not significantly different in these populations. Note that in this analysis, the population with microcalcifications did not present with isolated microcalcifications but with microcalcifications with or without other findings. In addition, the sensitivity is based on a mammogram assessment of 4 or 5 being positive, whereas an assessment of 1, 2, or 3 would be considered negative. The sensitivity increase of a mammogram assessment of 3 is considered positive; however, this is at the expense of specificity.

A more detailed look at the imaging features that guided interpretation in the IBMC study provides insight into how to improve MR imaging further as a diagnostic modality [24]. The initial decision in the interpretation of a diagnostic breast MR imaging scan is the detection of enhancement corresponding to the index finding (mammogram or clinical breast examination) that is leading to the diagnostic workup. In fact, the negative predictive value for enhancement of any type was 88% in the IBMC study, indicating that there were 12% of

cases in which no enhancement corresponding to the index lesion was reported and in which the ultimate diagnosis was cancer. This would suggest that MR imaging has a difficult time excluding cancer if a case of "no enhancement" can still turn out to be cancer. A closer look at these cases revealed that most of the cancers reported as nonenhancing were DCIS or lesions with mixed histology and small invasive components, however. In addition, all but one case presented with isolated microcalcifications (Fig. 2). Thus, it is clear that the lack of enhancement in the setting of isolated microcalcifications cannot exclude cancer. This makes sense, given the role of microcalcification as a sensitive biomarker for even microscopic disease that would not likely be detected by any macroscopic imaging technique. There was only a single case of architectural distortion that was associated with no reporting of enhancement on MR imaging that turned out to be invasive lobular cancer, however. Thus, the data would suggest that in the setting of a density or mass, the lack of enhancement on MR imaging may reliably exclude cancer.

The IBMC data offer further insight into the relative contributions of kinetic and architectural features in the interpretation of breast MR imaging. IBMC patients with enhancing abnormalities were invited back a second day for a standardized high-time resolution scan with identical imaging parameters across all sights. Compliance with the second scan was approximately 50%, and there was no obvious bias in the population that returned for the kinetic scan. Kinetic curves were extracted by readers from the most intensely enhancing portion of the lesion on the early postcontrast scans consistent with clinical standards. Quantitative and qualitative approaches to the kinetic data were tested. Qualitative assessment of the enhancement curve had the highest univariate model ROC area of 0.66. Of the quantitative kinetic features, the feature that best predicted diagnosis was the maximum enhancement rate, which had an ROC area of 0.64. Of note, 76% of kinetic curves that were described as wash-out were associated with a cancer diagnosis. In addition, 45% of curves that were described as persistent were also associated with a cancer diagnosis. This accounted for 28% of the cancers that underwent the kinetic study. Thus, although there is clearly diagnostic information in the kinetic curve, excluding cancer on the basis of a persistent enhancement curve alone would lead to false-negative findings. In a multivariate analysis, however, lesions with wash-out kinetics were approximately five times more likely to be cancer than those demonstrating persistent enhancement.

In terms of the architectural characteristics, for focal mass lesions, the qualitative enhancement

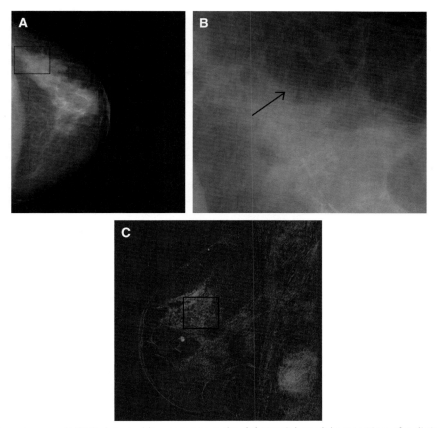

Fig. 2. MR imaging occult DCIS detected by mammography. (*A*) Cranial caudal projection of a digital mammogram of the left breast. (*B*) Magnification view of the lateral aspect demonstrates microcalcifications that underwent biopsy and demonstrated DCIS. (*C*) Subtraction MR imaging from the left breast with a box marking the expected area of the calcification demonstrates diffuse stippled enhancement without focal findings. This was a false-negative finding on MR imaging.

intensity (between 2 and 4 minutes after administration of contrast) and mass margin were the most important predictors of diagnosis. The smoother the margin and more weak the enhancement, the more likely the lesion was to be benign. In a multivariate analysis, spiculated lesions were approximately 18 to 20 times more likely to be cancer than smooth lesions. Intensely enhancing lesions were approximately 10 to 20 times more likely to be cancer than those demonstrating minimal enhancement. Rim enhancement also carried a 2 to 3 times higher risk of malignancy than not demonstrating rim enhancement.

With respect to nonmass enhancement, the distribution of enhancement was most predictive of diagnosis, with ductal and segmental distributions predicting malignancy and regional, patchy, and diffuse distributions predicting benignity. Enhancement intensity and form were the next most important features, respectively.

Practical implementation of MR imaging in the diagnostic setting

In any practical implementation of MR imaging in the diagnostic setting, the first rule of thumb is that the value of MR imaging in the setting of isolated mammogram microcalcifications is minimal. As tempting as it might be to use MR imaging to reduce concern over marginally suspicious calcification, clinical research experience does not support the use of MR imaging in this clinical setting. The decision to perform a biopsy of microcalcifications rests with mammography. The lesions that present as mammographic calcifications are exactly those lesions that have an admixture of normal stroma and epithelial tumor and are exactly those lesions that can represent false-negative cases on MR imaging. Although many of these cancers are detectable on MR imaging, the false-negative rate is high enough that you cannot rely on the absence of enhancement to exclude cancer. These lesions should undergo biopsy based on the level of mammographic suspicion. The only exception may be in the case of patchy or diffuse calcification, where the MR imaging may help to guide the biopsy site to maximize the likelihood of cancer detection in those cases in which localized suspicious enhancement is identified.

In contrast to the evaluation of mammographic microcalcifications, there are several scenarios in which MR imaging may represent a reasonable option for the workup of a finding on mammography. The first scenario is a mammographically detected mass. Most of these lesions ultimately represent cysts, fibroadenomas, intramammary lymph nodes, or a papilloma in the periareolar location. In most breast centers, directed ultrasound is the initial adjunctive imaging study of choice. The identification of a simple cyst places the lesions into BI-RADS category 2 (benign). If the lesion is found to be solid, several options are available. One option is ultrasound-guided biopsy. For those lesions that represent complex cysts, fine needle aspiration can

establish this diagnosis. For solid masses, core biopsy, which is minimally invasive, provides a definitive diagnosis, and eliminates the need for additional clinic visits in breast imaging centers in which the biopsy can be performed at the time of the diagnostic workup. As suggested previously, in those cases in which the sonographic features of a solid mass are all benign, imaging follow-up is considered a reasonable alternative to core biopsy [6]. In this setting, MR imaging may also be an alternative to core biopsy or short-term interval follow-up. Findings of high signal on T2 and lack of enhancement can definitively classify complex cystic lesions without requiring aspiration. In addition, fibroadenomas often have a fairly classic appearance, allowing an assessment of BI-RADS category 2 or 3 to be assigned to the lesion and avoiding biopsy. This scenario can be especially useful in patients with multiple solid masses in one or both breasts, where it may not be clear which, if any, mass should undergo tissue sampling.

Fibroadenomas may have several classic appearances on MR imaging. All fibroadenomas should

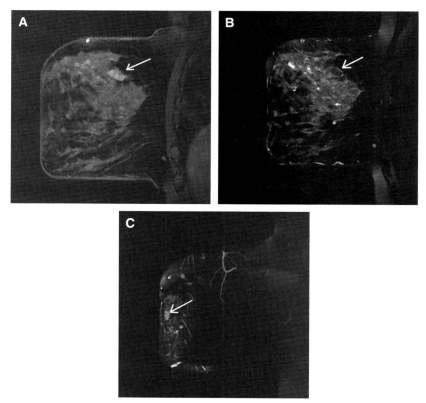

Fig. 3. (*A*) Postcontrast, 3D, spoiled gradient echo image demonstrates the classic oval shape, lobulated borders, and internal septations of a fibroadenoma. (*B*) T2-weighted image demonstrates the same fibroadenoma as a uniformly low signal intensity lesion typical of hyalinized fibroadenomas. (*C*) T2-weighted image of a different fibroadenoma in the same patient demonstrates a high-signal lesion with typical internal septation.

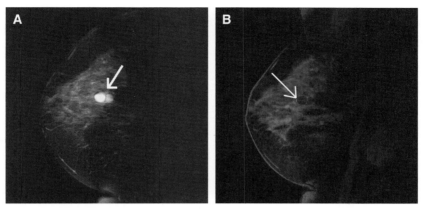

Fig. 4. Cyst. (*A*) T2-weighted image demonstrates a lobulated high-signal mass with internal septation. (*B*) Post-contrast scan demonstrates mild enhancement of a thin smooth rim and no contrast enhancement consistent with the diagnosis of a cyst.

have well-circumscribed margins. Most have a lobular shape, although some are round or oval. They often present with nonenhancing internal septations, giving the lesion a "cluster of grapes" appearance [25]. The T2-weighted intensity can vary from extremely bright to quite dark depending on the amount of glandular elements and hyalinization. It is not unusual for different lobules of a fibroadenoma to demonstrate different T2 signal intensity. The enhancement of fibroadenomas can also vary. They may not enhance at all, or they can enhance minimally or intensely. In addition, the different lobules of a fibroadenoma may enhance differently. Fibroadenomas that enhance intensely can also demonstrate wash-out kinetics. Given the variable appearance of fibroadenomas, a rational approach

needs to be taken to classify a lesion as a fibroadenoma on MR imaging.

To be classified as a fibroadenoma, lesions must be well circumscribed on all sequences, with smooth margins and a round or lobulated shape (Fig. 3). To classify the margins, if they are lobulated in shape, they must contain nonenhancing internal septations on T2-weighted or postcontrast images. If the entire lesion or one or more lobules of a lobulated lesion demonstrate low signal on T2-weighted images, this is supportive of fibroadenoma. If the entire lesion demonstrates high signal on T2-weighted images, it is also compatible with a fibroadenoma; however, a multiloculated cyst may have a similar appearance (Fig. 4). These diagnoses can be distinguished based on enhancement.

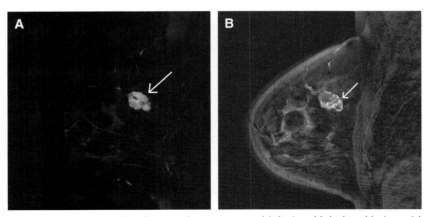

Fig. 5. Colloid carcinoma. (*A*) T2-weighted image demonstrates a high-signal lobulated lesion with internal septations, which represents colloid carcinoma in this case. (*B*) Postcontrast image demonstrates thick irregular rim enhancement of each lobule.

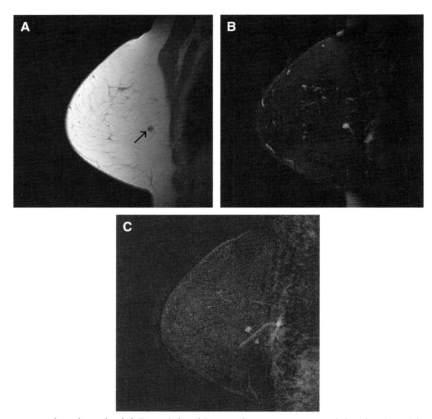

Fig. 6. Intramammary lymph node. (*A*) T1-weighted image demonstrates a nodular density with a small notch associated with a vascular pedicle typical of an intramammary lymph node. (*B*) T2-weighted image demonstrates the nodule to contain uniform high signal. (*C*) Postcontrast subtraction image demonstrates uniform intense enhancement.

The one pitfall is colloid cancers, which may have a lobulated shape, smooth margins, and internal septations. These lesions tend to have thickened enhancing rims, which can be used to distinguish them from fibroadenomas and cysts (Fig. 5).

Although many intramammary lymph nodes can be diagnosed on mammography, MR imaging can offer a definitive diagnosis in difficult cases. Lymph nodes are characterized by their location adjacent to a main blood vessel in the breast (Fig. 6), and their fatty hilum is best appreciated on the non–fat-suppressed T1-weighted images. They have the typical kidney bean shape with a fatty hilum. They also typically demonstrate high signal on T2-weighted images. They may demonstrate intense enhancement and often can have wash-out kinetics. This is a diagnosis that is based on lesion architecture.

Papillomas tend to be well-circumscribed masses and are typically 5 mm to 1 cm in size. Most often, they are located in the retroareolar portion of the breast, and the key to suggesting this diagnosis is identifying that the lesion is located within a breast duct. Given the risk of papillomas to contain cancer, it is usually suggested that these lesions undergo biopsy so that a diagnosis of papilloma may not avert a biopsy.

Another scenario in which MR imaging may be valuable is the mammographic asymmetric density. If the density is clearly identified on MR imaging, no architectural distortion is present, and the "density" demonstrates no contrast enhancement, its likelihood of being cancer is low, and it is reasonable to assess this finding as benign or probably benign.

Summary

The role of MR imaging as an adjunct in the diagnostic evaluation of findings on mammography or clinical examination continues to evolve. Clearly, the use of MR imaging to evaluate all suspicious screening findings is not reasonable or effective. In particular, the role of MR imaging in the setting of mammographic microcalcifications is limited. MR imaging may be used in cases of one or more mammographically detected masses or asymmetric density in an effort to avoid biopsy. Optimized MR imaging technique; careful mammography, ultrasound, and MR imaging correlation; and adherence to interpretation guidelines are important to avoid false-negative diagnoses.

References

[1] Humphrey LL, Helfand M, Chan BK, et al. Breast cancer screening: a summary of the evidence for the US Preventive Services Task Force. Ann Intern Med 2002;137:347–60.

[2] Institute of Medicine. Saving womens' lives: integration and innovation: a framework for progress in early detection and diagnosis of breast cancer. Washington (DC): National Academies Press; 2005.

[3] Fletcher SW, Elmore JG. Mammographic screening for breast cancer. N Engl J Med 2003;348: 1672–80.

[4] Hall FM, Storella JM, Silverstone DZ, et al. Nonpalpable breast lesions: recommendations for biopsy based on suspicion of carcinoma at mammography. Radiology 1988;167:353–8.

[5] Liberman L. Clinical management issues in percutaneous core breast biopsy. Radiol Clin North Am 2000;38(4):791–807.

[6] Stravos D, Thickman D, Rapp CL, et al. Solid breast nodules. Use of sonography to distinguish between benign and malignant lesions. Radiology 1995;96:123–34.

[7] Rosen EL, Turkington TG, Soo MS, et al. Detection of primary breast carcinoma with a dedicated, large-field-of-view FDG PET mammography device: initial experience. Radiology 2005;234(2):527–34.

[8] Mathieu I, Mazy S, Willemart B, et al. Inconclusive triple diagnosis in breast cancer imaging: is there a place for scintimammography? J Nucl Med 2005;46(10):1574–81.

[9] Kaiser WA, Zeitler E. MR imaging of the breast: fast imaging sequences with and without Gd-DTPA. Radiology 1989;170:681–6.

[10] Heywang SH, Wolf A, Pruss E, et al. MR imaging of the breast with Gd-DTPA: use and limitations. Radiology 1989;171:95–103.

[11] Harms SE, Flamig DP, Hesley KL, et al. MR imaging of the breast with rotating delivery of excitation off resonance: clinical experience with pathologic correlation. Radiology 1993;187: 493–501.

[12] Nunes LW, Schnall MD, Orel SG, et al. Breast MR imaging: interpretation model. Radiology 1997; 202:833–41.

[13] Boetes C, Barentsz JO, Mus RD, et al. MR characterization of suspicious breast lesions with a gadolinium-enhanced turboFLASH subtraction technique. Radiology 1994;193:777–81.

[14] Hulka CA, Smith BL, Sgroi DC, et al. Benign and malignant breast lesions: differentiation with echo-planar MR imaging. Radiology 1997;205: 33–8.

[15] Daniel BL, Yen YF, Glover GH, et al. Breast disease: dynamic spiral MR imaging. Radiology 1998;209(2):499–509.

[16] Schnall MD, Rosten S, Englander S, et al. A combined architectural and kinetic interpretation model for breast MR images. Acad Radiol 2001; 8(7):591–7.

[17] Kuhl CK, Mielcareck P, Klaschik S, et al. Dynamic breast MR imaging: are signal intensity time course data useful for differential diagnosis of enhancing lesions? Radiology 1999;211(1):101–10.

[18] Tofts PS, Berkowitz B, Schnall MD. Quantitative analysis of dynamic Gd-DTPA enhancement in breast tumors using a permeability model. Magn Reson Med 1995;33(4):564–8.

[19] Ikeda D, Hylton N, Kuhl C, et al. Breast imaging and reporting data system-magnetic resonance imaging in ACR BI-RADS-magnetic resonance, . ACR breast imaging and reporting data system, breast imaging atlas. Reston (VA): American College of Radiology; 2003.

[20] Song HK, Dougherty L, Schnall MD. Simultaneous acquisition of multiple resolution images for dynamic contrast enhanced imaging of the breast. Magn Reson Med 2001;46(3):503–9.

[21] Friedman PD, Swaminathan SV, Smith R. SENSE imaging of the breast. AJR Am J Roentgenol 2005;184(2):448–51.

[22] Kuhl CK, Schild HH, Morakkabati N. Dynamic bilateral contrast-enhanced MR imaging of the breast: trade-off between spatial and temporal resolution. Radiology 2005;236:789–800.

[23] Bluemke DA, Gatsonis CA, Chen MH, et al. Magnetic resonance imaging of the breast prior to biopsy. JAMA 2004;292(22):2735–42.

[24] Schnall MD, Blume J, Bluemke DA, et al. Diagnostic architectural and dynamic features at breast MR imaging: multicenter study. Radiology 2006;238(1):42–53.

[25] Hochman MG, Orel SG, Powell CM, et al. Fibroadenomas: MR imaging appearances with radiologic-histopathologic correlation. Radiology 1997;204(1):123–9.

MAGNETIC
RESONANCE
IMAGING CLINICS

Magn Reson Imaging Clin N Am 14 (2006) 339–349

Breast MR Imaging in Assessing Extent of Disease

Laura Liberman, MD[a,b,c],*

- Ipsilateral breast
  *MR imaging of the ipsilateral breast:
    Memorial Sloan-Kettering experience
  Involvement of skin, pectoral muscle,
    and chest wall*
- Contralateral breast
  *MR imaging of the contralateral breast:
    Memorial Sloan-Kettering experience*

- Ultrasonography versus MR imaging for
  extent of disease assessment
- Invasive lobular carcinoma
- Further investigation
- Summary
- References

To plan appropriate treatment for women with breast cancer, accurate assessment of extent of disease is necessary. Multifocal cancer (in multiple sites in one quadrant) indicates the need for wider excision than might otherwise be performed. Multicentric cancer (in more than one quadrant) usually precludes breast conservation and warrants mastectomy. Appropriate surgical planning also requires knowledge of involvement of the skin, pectoral muscle, or chest wall. Furthermore, identification of contralateral cancer indicates the need for contralateral breast surgery.

This chapter discusses the use of MR imaging in women with breast cancer to evaluate extent of disease in the ipsilateral breast (including multifocality and multicentricity, skin, pectoral muscle, or chest wall involvement) and the contralateral breast. It also compares ultrasonography and MR imaging in extent of disease assessment, and discusses the use of MR imaging in women with invasive lobular cancer. Avenues for future study are

explored, including identification of subgroups of women most likely to benefit from the use of breast MR imaging in assessing extent of disease and the potential survival benefit of breast MR imaging in this scenario. The need for the capability to perform biopsy of lesions detected by MR imaging only is emphasized.

Ipsilateral breast

Pathology findings suggest that women with one area of proven breast cancer may have additional sites of cancer in the ipsilateral breast [1,2]. Pathologic analyses of mastectomy specimens have found sites of cancer other than the index cancer in the ipsilateral breast in 20% to 63%. Among these additional sites of cancer, 19% to 67% were invasive. In 20% to 47% of mastectomy specimens, additional sites of cancer were in quadrants different from that of the index lesion and therefore

[a] Breast Imaging Section, Memorial Sloan-Kettering Cancer Center, 1275 York Avenue, New York, NY 10021, USA
[b] Department of Radiology, Memorial Hospital, New York, NY 10021, USA
[c] Department of Radiology, Weill Medical College of Cornell University, New York, NY 10021, USA
* Breast Imaging Section, Memorial Sloan-Kettering Cancer Center, 1275 York Avenue, New York, NY 10021.
E-mail address: libermal@mskcc.org

doi:10.1016/j.mric.2006.07.007

represented multicentric disease. In women who had ductal carcinoma in situ (DCIS) treated with mastectomy, a multifocal distribution with gaps larger than 1 cm was identified in 8%, and DCIS involved more than one quadrant in 23% to 47%. Women with DCIS measuring 2.5 cm or larger had the highest likelihood of cancer outside the index quadrant [1,2].

In prior investigations of women with invasive breast cancer who had breast-conserving surgery, local recurrence rates at 15-year follow-up were 36% without radiation and 12% with radiation [3]; in a more recent study, the local recurrence rate 20 years after lumpectomy and radiation for invasive cancer was 9% [4]. In prior studies of women with DCIS who had breast-conserving surgery, local recurrence rates at 6-year follow-up were 21% without radiation and 10% with radiation [5]; local recurrence rates at 8-year follow-up were 31% without radiation and 13% with radiation [6]; and local recurrence rate at 15-year follow-up was 19% with radiation [7]. The local recurrence rates greater than 20% without radiation are within the 20% to 63% range of additional sites of cancer reported in the pathology studies [2]. The lower frequency of local recurrence after irradiation suggests that radiation destroys or slows the growth of some of these sites of disease.

In prior investigations, MR imaging identified additional sites of ipsilateral cancer that were not identified on mammography or physical examination in 16% (range, 6%–34%) of women who have breast cancer [2,8–15]. Additional sites of cancer in the same quadrant as the index cancer (multifocal sites of disease) were found in 1% to 20% of women (Fig. 1), and additional sites of cancer in different quadrants from the index cancer (multicentric sites of disease) were found in 2% to 24% of women (Fig. 2) [2,8–10,12–15].

Preoperative identification of additional sites of cancer may allow their removal and could lower the frequency of local recurrence. Furthermore, MR imaging–guided resection of these additional sites could reduce the need for postoperative radiation therapy. Validation of these hypotheses requires further study.

MR imaging of the ipsilateral breast: Memorial Sloan-Kettering experience

In a study from our institution of 70 women with percutaneously proven breast cancer who were considering breast conservation, biopsy was recommended for MR imaging–detected ipsilateral lesions in 51% of women [2]. The positive predictive value (PPV) of biopsy was 52% and was higher for lesions in the same quadrant as the index cancer

as compared with different quadrants (64% versus 31%, $P = .07$). The 52% PPV of biopsy is within the 18% to 88% range of PPVs for biopsies based on MR imaging findings in high-risk women [16–18] and higher than the 20% to 40% range of PPVs for mammographically guided needle localization and surgical excision in the general population [19].

In this study, additional sites of cancer in the ipsilateral breast were identified by MR imaging in 19 (27%) of 70 women with percutaneously diagnosed breast cancer [2]. Additional sites of cancer in were invasive in 11 (16%) of 70 women and DCIS in eight (11%) of 70 women. Location of additional sites of cancer with respect to the index tumor was in the same quadrant in 14 (20%) of 70 women, in a different quadrant in three (4%) women, and in both the same and different quadrants in two (3%) women. MR imaging detected ipsilateral lesions that were benign in 17 (24%) of 70 women. Changes owing to prior percutaneous biopsy were infrequent during MR imaging and did not interfere with MR imaging interpretation. Postbiopsy changes observed included a clip in 12 (17%) women and small hematoma in two; no skin thickening, skin enhancement, or needle tracts were identified.

The 27% frequency of finding additional sites of cancer by MR imaging is within the 6% to 34% range of ipsilateral MRI-detected cancers in the published literature and within the 20% to 63% range of frequencies of additional sites of cancer reported in previous studies that performed pathologic analyses of mastectomy specimens [2]. The frequency with which MR imaging depicted additional sites of cancer in the ipsilateral breast was higher in women with rather than without a family history of breast cancer (14 of 33 = 42% versus 5 of 37 = 14%; $P < .02$) and in women in whom the index tumor was invasive lobular carcinoma rather than other histologies (6 of 11 = 55% versus 13 of 70 = 19%; $P < .06$).

Among women who had additional ipsilateral sites of cancer detected by MR imaging in our study, the additional sites of cancer were in the same quadrant as the index cancer in approximately three quarters (74%) and in quadrants other than the index cancer in approximately one quarter (26%) [2]. This distribution of additional sites of cancer detected by MR imaging is similar to the distribution of local recurrences at 15-year follow-up of women with invasive breast cancer who had breast conservation (75% in the same quadrant and 25% in different quadrants than the index tumor) [3]. This finding suggests, but does not prove, that the additional sites detected by MR imaging may have biological relevance.

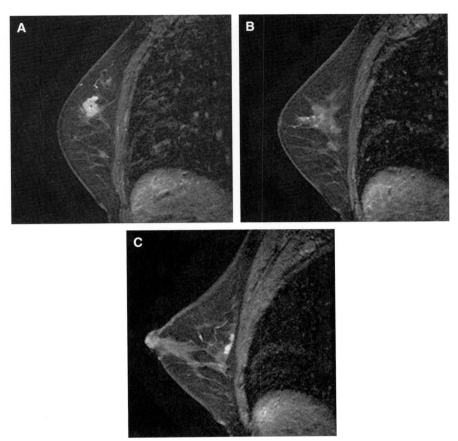

Fig. 1. 37-year-old woman with palpable mass right breast upper inner quadrant identified on mammography and sonography (not shown), for which core biopsy results showed invasive ductal carcinoma, poorly differentiated, and DCIS. (*A*) Sagittal, fat-suppressed, T$_1$-weighted, contrast-enhanced image from MR image of the right (ipsilateral) breast shows a lobulated, heterogeneously enhancing mass measuring up to 1.8 cm, corresponding to the biopsy-proven cancer. Surgical excision found 1.7-cm invasive ductal carcinoma and DCIS. Sentinel nodes were negative. (*B*) Sagittal, fat-suppressed, T$_1$-weighted, contrast-enhanced image from MR image of the right (ipsilateral) breast shows clumped ductal enhancement extending anteriorly from the mass toward the nipple in the same quadrant. MR imaging–guided needle localization and surgical excision yielded DCIS, solid, cribriform, and flat, with high nuclear grade and extensive necrosis. (*C*) Sagittal, fat-suppressed, T$_1$-weighted, contrast-enhanced image from MR image of the right (ipsilateral) breast shows focal clumped enhancement posteriorly, in approximately the 9:00 axis, a different quadrant. MR image–guided localization for surgical excision yielded DCIS, solid, cribriform, and flat, with high nuclear grade and moderate necrosis, confirming the presence of multicentric disease, for which mastectomy was performed.

Involvement of skin, pectoral muscle, and chest wall

Breast MR imaging may be helpful in assessment of skin involvement. MR imaging–depicted skin enhancement may identify a site for biopsy or assist the surgeon in excising the area of concern [20] (Fig. 2). Inflammatory carcinoma, characterized histologically by tumor involvement of the dermal lymphatics, produces skin induration. Breast MR imaging in inflammatory carcinoma may show focal or diffuse enhancement of the thickened skin, a pattern that may also be seen in mastitis [20].

Rieber and coauthors [21] reported skin thickening that was bright on T$_2$-weighted images and medium intensity on T$_1$-weighted images in 90% of patients who had inflammatory carcinoma versus 55% of patients who had mastitis. The sensitivity and specificity of breast MR imaging in assessing skin involvement requires further investigation.

Breast MR imaging may be valuable in evaluating masses that are posterior in location [22]. Involvement of the pectoral muscle or chest wall impacts surgical treatment. Superficial invasion of the muscle may require excision of a portion of the muscle, invasion of the full thickness of the muscle may

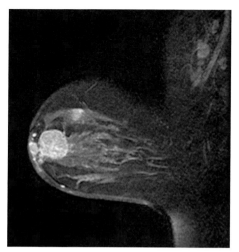

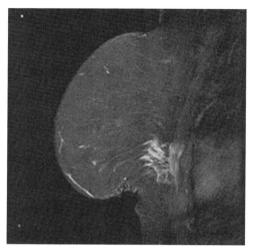

Fig. 2. 31-year-old woman with palpable, mammographically and sonographically evident mass in the left breast, retroareolar region, for which ultrasound-guided core biopsy showed poorly differentiated invasive ductal carcinoma with vascular invasion. Sagittal, T_1-weighted, contrast-enhanced image from MR imaging of the left breast shows the index cancer, a smaller satellite lesion superoposteriorly, suspicious axillary adenopathy, and a skin nodule anterior to the index cancer. Core biopsy of the satellite nodule yielded poorly differentiated invasive ductal carcinoma. Ultrasound-guided, fine-needle aspiration of the left axillary adenopathy was positive for malignant cells. Core biopsy of the skin nodule showed invasive ductal carcinoma, poorly differentiated, involving the deep dermis. The patient is being treated with preoperative chemotherapy.

Fig. 3. 64-year-old woman with palpable mass left breast lower inner quadrant identified at mammography and sonography, for which core biopsy yielded invasive ductal carcinoma. Sagittal, fat-suppressed, T_1-weighted, contrast enhancement image shows spiculated mass posteriorly in the left breast lower inner quadrant, corresponding to biopsy-proven cancer. Enhancement extends through the full thickness of the pectoral muscle, indicating pectoral muscle invasion, but does not involve the intercostal muscles. The patient had preoperative chemotherapy followed by mastectomy, including removal of the pectoral muscle. Surgical histology yielded invasive ductal carcinoma involving breast, skeletal muscle, and fibroadipose tissue, with clear margins of resection, and negative axillary nodes.

necessitate radical mastectomy, and involvement of the chest wall (ribs, intercostals muscles, serratus anterior muscle) may warrant chest wall resection [20]. Mammography and physical examination often provide incomplete information regarding these posterior structures.

In a study from our institution, Morris and colleagues [22] reported on 19 women who had posterior enhancing breast masses at preoperative breast MR imaging. Five (26%) of these 19 women had masses that abutted the muscle with obliteration of the fat plane and muscle enhancement; all five had muscle involvement at surgery (Fig. 3). In the remaining 14 (74%) patients, no enhancement of muscle was seen; none of these had invasion of the muscle at surgery. The investigators concluded that violation of the fat plane without other findings did not indicate muscle or chest wall involvement; extension of tumor into underlying muscle or chest wall was indicated by abnormal enhancement within these deep structures [22].

Contralateral breast

The contralateral breast is at high risk in women who have breast cancer. A synchronous contralateral cancer, variably defined as occurring within 3 months, 6 months, or 1 year after diagnosis of the index cancer, is found by mammography, physical examination, or both in approximately 2% of women who have breast cancer. Women with synchronous bilateral breast cancer are more likely to have a genetic predisposition to breast cancer and multicentric disease in the index cancer; they also have a trend toward decreased local control and overall survival [23]. For women with unilateral breast cancer, a subsequent (metachronous) contralateral cancer develops in 0.5% to 1.0% per year, with a lifetime risk of 15%. Among metachronous contralateral breast cancers, 16% metastasize and 7% are lethal.

Management options for the asymptomatic contralateral breast have included close observation, blind contralateral biopsy, chemoprevention, and prophylactic mastectomy [23]. Now, breast MR imaging may be used to evaluate the contralateral breast in women who have known breast cancer. In prior studies, MR imaging detected an otherwise occult cancer in the contralateral breast in 6% (range, 3%–24%) [12,23–26]. This frequency should be interpreted in the context of the likelihood of detecting cancer at high-risk MR imaging screening, reported as 4% (range, 2%–7%) [16–18].

MR imaging of the contralateral breast: Memorial Sloan-Kettering experience

In a study of 223 women with breast cancer who had contralateral breast MRI at our institution, contralateral breast biopsy was recommended in 72 (32%) women and performed in 61 women [23]. Cancer not identified at mammography and physical examination was depicted by MR imaging in 12 women, constituting 20% (12 of 61) women who had contralateral biopsy and 5% (12 of 223) women who had contralateral breast MR imaging. Among these 12 cancers, six (50%) were DCIS and six (50%) were invasive (median size, 0.5 cm; range, 0.1–1.0 cm). Contralateral biopsy found benign (n = 31) or high-risk (n = 18) lesions in 49 women, constituting 80% of the women who had contralateral biopsy and 22% of the women who had contralateral breast MR imaging.

MR imaging depicted an otherwise unsuspected contralateral cancer in 5% of women who had breast cancer in our study (Fig. 4). The likelihood of MR imaging depicting an otherwise unsuspected contralateral breast cancer was higher in women with rather than without a family history of breast cancer in a first-degree relative (13% versus 3%, $P = .02$) and in women whose index tumor was invasive lobular rather than other histologies (13% versus 4%, $P < .07$). The 5% frequency of depicting contralateral breast cancer by MR imaging in our study does not differ significantly ($P = .12$) from the 3% (26 of 871) prevalence of cancer at blind contralateral upper outer quadrant in a prior report by Cody [28]. However, all of the patients in Cody's study had contralateral breast biopsy [28]; in our study, MR imaging facilitated diagnosis of these contralateral cancers while only requiring biopsy in one third (32%) of women.

In our study, cancer was found in 20% of women who had contralateral breast biopsy based on MR imaging [23]. This PPV is lower than the 47% to 80% range of those previously reported for biopsy based on MR imaging findings in the contralateral breast in women who had known breast cancer [24,25,27] and at the low end of the 18% to 89% range of PPVs reported for biopsy based on MR imaging findings in women at high risk for breast cancer [16,17]. The 20% PPV is also at the low end of the 20% to 40% range for mammographically guided needle localization and surgical excision in the general population [19].

Our data suggest that MR imaging of the contralateral breast may have a potentially disturbing consequence. In our study, prophylactic contralateral mastectomy was performed in 5% of our women. The frequency of prophylactic mastectomy was

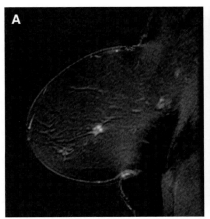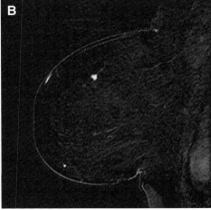

Fig. 4. 74-year-old asymptomatic woman with mammographically detected mass in the right breast, 9:00 axis. Ultrasound-guided core biopsy yielded invasive lobular carcinoma. (*A*) Sagittal, T_1-weighted, contrast-enhanced, subtraction image from MR imaging of the right (ipsilateral) breast shows a spiculated, heterogeneous and rim-enhancing mass consistent with the patient's biopsy-proven cancer. Lumpectomy and sentinel node biopsy were performed, yielding invasive lobular carcinoma with negative sentinel nodes. (*B*) Sagittal, T_1-weighted, contrast-enhanced, subtraction image from MR image of the left (contralateral) breast shows an intensely enhancing lobulated, smooth mass, without mammographic or sonographic correlate. Delayed images (not shown) demonstrated washout. MR image–guided needle localization yielded invasive ductal carcinoma, 0.6 cm, with sentinel node micrometastases. The patient had breast-conserving surgery.

higher in women in whom a biopsy was recommended based on MR imaging than among women who were not referred for biopsy (9% versus 3%, $P = .11$). Identification of an abnormality at breast MR imaging may have contributed to the patient's decision to have a prophylactic contralateral mastectomy. Prophylactic mastectomy may be a reasonable choice, but women and the doctors caring for them should be aware of the limited specificity of MR imaging to make an informed decision [29]; at our center, 80% of biopsies performed for MR imaging–depicted contralateral breast lesions yielded benign results.

Ultrasonography versus MR imaging for extent of disease assessment

Breast ultrasonography can depict additional sites of cancer in women who have breast cancer [30–34], but breast MR imaging may have higher sensitivity in this scenario. The accuracies of MR imaging, mammography, and ultrasonography were assessed by Boetes and coauthors [32] in a study of 61 cancers in 60 women who were having mastectomy. Of the additional invasive cancers, 31% were depicted by mammography, 38% by ultrasound scan, and 100% by MR imaging.

A comparison of whole-breast ultrasonography and MR imaging as adjuncts to mammography in 101 women who had breast cancer was performed by Hlawatsch and colleagues [33]. Pathologic analysis found multifocal or multicentric invasive cancer in 27 tumors. Of these 27, 48% were diagnosed correctly by mammography alone, 63% by a combination of mammography and ultrasonography, and 81% by MR imaging. Nine of the index cancers were not visible at mammography but were seen at ultrasound scan. Use of ultrasonography benefited 13 women and yielded false-positive results in two. Use of MR imaging benefited seven women and produced false-positive results in eight.

Berg and coworkers [35] compared mammography, ultrasonography, and MR imaging in 177 malignant foci in 121 cancerous breasts. MR imaging depicted 105 (95%) of 110 foci of invasive ductal carcinoma, 28 (96%) of 29 foci of invasive lobular carcinoma, and 34 (89%) of 38 cases of DCIS. MR imaging showed higher sensitivity than mammography for all tumor types ($P < .01$) and higher sensitivity than ultrasonography for DCIS ($P < .001$). After combined physical examination, mammography, and ultrasonography, MR imaging depicted additional tumor in 12 (12%) of 96 breasts and led to overestimation of extent of disease in another six (6%); ultrasound scans showed no detection benefit after MR imaging. Contralateral breast cancer was identified in 10 (9%) of 111 patients. Method

of detection of contralateral breast cancer was mammography in six, ultrasonography and MR imaging in three, and clinical examination only in one.

Data regarding extent of disease assessment should be interpreted in conjunction with other published data comparing breast ultrasound scan and MR imaging. Studies of high-risk women who were screened with mammography, ultrasonography, and MR imaging reported sensitivities of 77% to 100% for MR imaging versus 33% to 43% for ultrasonography [36–38]. MR imaging is more sensitive than ultrasonography in the detection of DCIS [30]. The 18% to 89% PPV of biopsy in studies of MR imaging screening [16–18] is significantly higher than the 9% to 16% PPV of biopsy in studies of screening breast ultrasound scan [39]. Ultrasonography, however, is faster, less expensive, widely available, and provides ready access for biopsies. Both MR imaging and ultrasonography may yield false-positive results, with the proportion of false-positives depending on the patient population, technique, and operator experience. Additional study comparing MR imaging and ultrasound in assessing extent of disease would be valuable.

Invasive lobular carcinoma

Invasive lobular cancer accounts for approximately 10% to 14% of invasive breast carcinomas [40]. The mammogram often is more falsely negative in invasive lobular than in invasive ductal cancer because of the tendency of the cells to grow in a single file arrangement, usually without calcification. Invasive lobular cancer also may have a higher frequency of multicentricity and bilaterality than invasive ductal cancer [45]. Breast MR imaging shows a variety of enhancement patterns in invasive lobular cancer and may be useful in assessment of extent of disease in these women [41–45].

Correlation of MR imaging and mammography in the ipsilateral breast was performed by Rodenko and colleagues [43] in a study of 20 women who had invasive lobular cancer. The correlation between imaging and pathologic extent of disease was higher for breast MR imaging than for mammography (85% versus 32%; $P < .0001$). MR imaging correctly classified all nine multicentric cases (100%) and overestimated two of 11 unicentric cases (18%). Mammography incorrectly classified all seven multicentric cases as unicentric disease; in one woman classified as having multicentric disease by mammography, pathologic analysis found unicentric disease [43].

A review of ipsilateral MR imaging and pathology findings was performed by Weinstein and coauthors [44] in a study of 32 women who had invasive lobular cancer. MR imaging showed more extensive tumor than conventional imaging studies and affected clinical management in half of the women. Among 18 women who did not have excisional biopsy before MR imaging, MR imaging was equal to mammography and sonography in predicting extent of disease in 10 (56%) and superior in eight (44%). MR imaging patterns of invasive lobular cancer in these 18 women were spiculated or irregular mass (n = 10), regional or multifocal enhancement (n = 7), or regional enhancement and architectural distortion (n = 1).

The preoperative MR imaging findings of 19 women who had invasive lobular cancer were reviewed by Yeh and coworkers [45]. They reported focal heterogeneously enhancing mass in eight (42%), regional enhancement in five (26%), and other patterns in six (32%). Among eight focal masses, margins were ill defined in six and spiculated in two; shape was irregular in seven and round in one. In 15 cases, the investigators evaluated the extraction flow (EF) product, a quantitative measure of gadolinium uptake over time. Peak EFs in these 15 invasive lobular cancers ranged from 25 to 120, with normal tissue threshold EF level less than or equal to 25; most tumors had EFs in the 30s. MR imaging depicted four cases of multifocal disease and one case of unsuspected contralateral disease.

In a study from our institution, Quan and colleagues [42] evaluated the impact of breast MR imaging on surgical treatment in 62 women with invasive lobular carcinoma. Among 51 women who had ipsilateral breast MR imaging, biopsy was recommended in 19 (37%) and yielded a cancer separate from the index tumor in 11 women, constituting 58% (11 of 19) women who had ipsilateral biopsy and 22% (11 of 51) women who had ipsilateral breast MR imaging (Fig. 5). In these 11 ipsilateral cancers, histologic findings were invasive lobular carcinoma in ten and DCIS in one. Among 53 women who had contralateral breast MRI, biopsy was recommended in 20 (38%) and led to detection of cancer in five women, constituting 25% (5 of 20) women who had contralateral biopsy and 9% (5 of 53) women who had contralateral breast MRI. Among five contralateral breast cancers, three were invasive (ductal in two and lobular in one) and two were DCIS.

These findings show that breast MR imaging has a high likelihood of depicting more than one site of cancer in women who have invasive lobular cancer. In our institution, breast MR imaging was more likely to identify additional sites of ipsilateral and contralateral cancer in women whose index tumor was invasive lobular carcinoma rather than other histologies [2,23]. The frequency with which MR

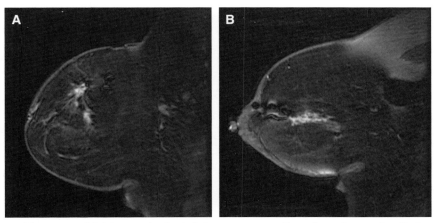

Fig. 5. 78-year-old woman with history of prior left lumpectomy, axillary dissection, and radiation for invasive cancer and prior right breast biopsy yielding lobular carcinoma in situ (LCIS). Mammogram (not shown) showed new distortion in the right breast, for which ultrasound-guided core biopsy yielded invasive lobular carcinoma. (*A*) Sagittal, fat-suppressed, T_1-weighted, contrast-enhanced image from MR imaging of the right (ipsilateral) breast shows two spiculated masses in the right breast upper outer quadrant, one of which had undergone core biopsy yielding invasive lobular cancer. Surgery found multifocal invasive lobular cancer, ranging from 0.5 to 1.6 cm, and DCIS, solid, intermediate nuclear grade, with minimal necrosis. Sentinel nodes were free of tumor. (*B*) Sagittal, fat-suppressed, T_1-weighted, contrast-enhanced image from MR imaging of the left (contralateral) breast shows ductal clumped enhancement posterior to the surgical clips from prior lumpectomy. MR image–guided needle localization yielded invasive ductal carcinoma, 0.5 cm, and DCIS, cribriform and flat, with high nuclear grade and moderate necrosis. The patient had bilateral mastectomies.

imaging depicts additional sites of cancer is higher in the ipsilateral than the contralateral breast. In women with invasive lobular cancer in whom MR imaging identifies additional suspicious areas, as in women with other cancer histologies, biopsy is necessary for tissue diagnosis.

Further investigation

Published studies have found that in women who have breast cancer, breast MR imaging can identify additional sites of cancer in the ipsilateral and contralateral breast and can identify involvement of the skin, pectoral muscle, and chest wall. The use of breast MR imaging in assessing extent of disease in the breasts may be useful, but further work is necessary. It would be valuable to identify specific subgroups of women with breast cancer in whom MR imaging is most likely to identify otherwise unsuspected sites of cancer. These subgroups could include specific patient factors such as specific risk factors, history (eg, prior breast cancer), breast parenchymal density, menopausal status, or cancer histology (such as invasive lobular cancer). At our institution, for example, we found that the likelihood of finding additional sites of cancer with MR imaging in the ipsilateral breast was higher in women who have invasive lobular histology in the index cancer and in women who have a family history of breast cancer; the likelihood of finding contralateral cancer was higher in women who had invasive lobular histology and in women who had a family history of breast cancer in a first-degree relative. Additional studies, with larger numbers of women and multivariate statistical analysis [46], are needed.

The published data suggest that in the ipsilateral breast, most additional sites of cancer depicted at breast MRI are in the same quadrant as the index cancer. These findings are consistent with the pathology data, in which most additional sites of cancer are in the same quadrant as the index tumor, and the clinical follow-up data, in which most recurrences occur in the same quadrant as the original cancer. For those women who have multifocal cancer (involving multiple areas in the same quadrant), excision of the entire quadrant as the initial therapeutic surgery could potentially remove all sites of disease. Quadrantectomy, which has been studied extensively and performed in Europe [47], is less frequently performed in the United States. The MR imaging experience suggests that quadrantectomy as the initial therapeutic surgery in breast conservation may warrant reconsideration.

An important unanswered question is whether the use of breast MR imaging in assessing extent of disease improves disease-free or overall survival rates. Is the MR imaging depicting disease that would be indolent or controlled by radiation, thus leading us to perform more aggressive surgery than necessary? This question could be addressed in a trial in which women who have breast cancer are assigned randomly to undergo or not undergo breast MR imaging examination before definitive surgery, with long-term follow-up data to assess disease-free and overall survival rates. Such a trial may be logistically and ethically challenging in an era in which breast MR imaging is available for clinical use. Furthermore, many interventions in medicine are performed without randomized, controlled trials showing mortality benefit, including our screening recommendations for women at high genetic risk of breast cancer and the performance of diagnostic mammography.

In the absence of data from randomized, controlled trials, the US Preventive Services Task Force states that management recommendations may appropriately be based on other sources, such as observational studies, data extrapolation, and expert opinion [48]. Published data in the literature indicate that the 16% frequency of identifying additional sites of cancer in the ipsilateral breast by MR imaging is within the 9% to 19% range of local recurrences at 15- 20-year follow-up after breast conservation with radiation. The distribution of additional sites of cancer identified by MR imaging (most of which are in the same quadrant as the index cancer) parallels the distribution of local recurrences. These data suggest that the additional sites of cancer depicted by MR imaging may be of biological significance, although the data do not prove a survival benefit.

If breast MR imaging is performed in the extent of disease setting, several caveats should be remembered. Not all biopsies performed for MR imaging–detected lesions yield cancer. At our institution, for example, half of the biopsies in the ipsilateral breast and 80% of the biopsies in the contralateral breast are benign. Mastectomy should not be recommended based on MR imaging findings alone; biopsy is necessary for tissue diagnosis. Among MR imaging–detected lesions referred for biopsy, ultrasonography fails to show a correlate in up to 77% [49]. If breast MR imaging is used in the assessment of extent of disease, it is necessary to have the capability to perform biopsy of lesions detected by MR imaging only [50–52]. Finally, additional biopsies (particularly if performed with surgery) may compromise the cosmetic result of breast conservation. Improving the specificity of breast MR imaging by research into the imaging–histologic correlation and promising techniques such as MR imaging spectroscopy [53,54] may prove valuable in this regard.

Summary

Planning appropriate surgical treatment for women who have breast cancer requires accurate assessment of extent of disease. MR imaging can depict breast cancer that is not palpable and not evident at mammography or ultrasonography. Among women with breast cancer who had breast MR imaging for assessment of extent of disease in published studies, MR imaging depicted an otherwise unsuspected cancer in the ipsilateral breast in 16% (range, 6%–34%) and in the contralateral breast in 6% (range, 3%–24%). MR imaging is most likely to identify additional sites of disease in the ipsilateral and contralateral breast in women with invasive lobular histology in the index cancer and a family history of breast cancer. MR imaging can also assist in the evaluating involvement of the skin, pectoral muscle, and chest wall.

Although published data indicate that breast MR imaging can depict additional sites of cancer in women with breast cancer, further investigation is necessary. In which subgroups of women, based on patient, breast, or lesion factors, is MR imaging most likely to identify additional sites of cancer? Does identification of these additional sites improve disease-free or overall survival? A randomized, controlled trial would provide information, but the need for and logistics of such a study remain a matter of debate. Potential disadvantages of MR imaging include cost and additional procedures, such as follow-up and biopsy. Furthermore, for breast MR imaging to be useful in assessing extent of disease, it is necessary to have the capability to perform biopsy of lesions identified only by MR imaging. Additional work, including refinement of criteria and methods for performing biopsy of MR imaging–detected lesions and long-term follow-up evaluation, is essential to optimize the use of breast MR imaging in assessing the extent of disease.

References

[1] Liberman L. Assessment of extent of disease using magnetic resonance imaging. In: Morris EA, Liberman L, editors. Breast MRI: diagnosis and intervention. New York: Springer, Inc.; 2005. p. 200–13.

[2] Liberman L, Morris EA, Dershaw DD, et al. MR imaging of the ipsilateral breast in women with percutaneously proven breast cancer. AJR 2003; 180:901–10.

[3] Fisher ER, Anderson S, Tan-Chiu E, et al. Fifteen-year prognostic discriminants for invasive breast carcinoma: National Surgical Adjuvant Breast and Bowel Project Protocol-06. Cancer 2001;91: 1679–87.

[4] Veronesi U, Cascinelli N, Mariani L, et al. Twenty-year follow-up of a randomized study comparing breast-conserving surgery with radical mastectomy for early breast cancer. N Engl J Med 2002;347:1227–32.

[5] Van Zee KJ, Liberman L, Samli B, et al. Long term follow-up of women with ductal carcinoma in situ treated with breast conserving surgery. Cancer 1999;86:1757–67.

[6] Fisher ER, Dignam J, Tan-Chiu E, et al. Pathologic findings from the National Surgical Adjuvant Breast Project (NSABP) eight-year update of Protocol B-17: intraductal carcinoma. Cancer 1999; 86:429–38.

[7] Solin LJ, Kurtz J, Fourquet A, et al. Fifteen-year results of breast-conserving surgery and definitive breast irradiation for the treatment of ductal carcinoma in situ of the breast. J Clin Oncol 1996; 14:754–63.

[8] Bedrosian I, Schlencker J, Spitz FR, et al. Magnetic resonance imaging-guided biopsy of mammographically and clinically occult breast lesions. Ann Surg Oncol 2002;9:457–61.

[9] Boetes C, Mus RDM, Holland R, et al. Breast tumors: comparative accuracy of MR imaging relative to mammography and US for demonstrating extent. Radiology 1995;197:743–7.

[10] Drew P, Chatterjee S, Turnbull L, et al. Dynamic contrast-enhanced magnetic resonance imaging of the breast is superior to triple assessment for the pre-operative detection of multifocal breast cancer. Ann Surg Oncol 1999;5: 599–603.

[11] Esserman L, Hylton NM, Yassa L, et al. Utility of magnetic resonance imaging in the management of breast cancer: evidence for improved preoperative staging. J Clin Oncol 1999;17:110–9.

[12] Fischer U, Kopka L, Grabbe E. Breast carcinoma: effect of preoperative contrast-enhanced MR imaging on the therapeutic approach. Radiology 1999;213:881–8.

[13] Harms SE, Flamig DP, Hesley KL, et al. MR imaging of the breast with rotating delivery of excitation off resonance: clinical experience with pathologic correlation. Radiology 1993;187:493–501.

[14] Mumtaz H, Hall-Craggs MA, Davidson T, et al. Staging of symptomatic primary breast cancer with MR imaging. AJR 1997;169:417–24.

[15] Orel SG, Schnall MD, Powell CM, et al. Staging of suspected breast cancer: effect of MR imaging and MR-guided biopsy. Radiology 1995;196: 115–22.

[16] Liberman L. Breast cancer screening with MRI: what are the data for patients at high risk? N Engl J Med 2004;351:497–500.

[17] Liberman L. The high-risk patient and magnetic resonance imaging. In: Morris EA, Liberman L, editors. Breast MRI: Diagnosis and intervention. New York: Springer, Inc.; 2005. p. 184–99.

[18] Morris EA, Liberman L, Ballon DJ, et al. MRI of occult breast carcinoma in a high-risk population. AJR 2003;181:619–26.

[19] Jackman RJ, Marzoni FA. Needle-localized breast biopsy: why do we fail? Radiology 1997;204: 677–84.

[20] Morris EA. Cancer staging with breast MR imaging. In: Schnall MD, Orel SG, editors. Breast MR Imaging. Philadelphia: WB Saunders; 2001. p. 333–44.

[21] Rieber A, Tomczak RJ, Mergo PJ, et al. MRI of the breast in the differential diagnosis of mastitis versus inflammatory carcinoma and follow-up. J Comput Assist Tomogr 1997;21:128–32.

[22] Morris EA, Schwartz LH, Drotman MB, et al. Evaluation of pectoralis major muscle in patients with posterior breast tumors on breast MRI: early experience. Radiology 2000;214: 67–72.

[23] Liberman L, Morris EA, Kim CM, et al. MR imaging findings in the contralateral breast in women with recently diagnosed breast cancer. AJR 2003; 180:333–41.

[24] Kuhl CK, Schmiedel A, Morakkabati N, et al. Breast MR imaging of the asymptomatic contralateral breast in the work-up or follow-up of patients with unilateral breast cancer [abstract]. Radiology 2000;217(P):268.

[25] Lee SG, Orel SG, Woo IJ, et al. MR imaging screening of the contralateral breast in patients with newly diagnosed breast cancer: preliminary results. Radiology 2003;226:773–8.

[26] Rieber A, Tomczak R, Merkle E, et al. MRI of histologically confirmed mammary carcinoma: clinical relevance of diagnostic procedures for detection of multifocal or contralateral secondary carcinoma [abstract]. Am J Roentgenol 1998;170(Suppl):48–9.

[27] Slanetz PJ, Edmister WB, Yeh ED, et al. Occult contralateral breast carcinoma incidentally detected by breast magnetic resonance imaging. Breast J 2002;8:145–8.

[28] Cody HS. Routine contralateral breast biopsy: helpful or irrelevant? Ann Surg 1997;225: 370–6.

[29] Montgomery LL, Tran KN, Heelan MC, et al. Issues of regret in women with contralateral prophylactic mastectomies. Ann Surg Oncol 1999; 6:546–52.

[30] Berg WA, Gilbreath PL. Multicentric and multifocal cancer: whole-breast US in preoperative evaluation. Radiology 2000;214:59–66.

[31] Berg WA, Nguyen TK, Gutierrez L, et al. Local extent of disease: preoperative evaluation of the breast cancer patient with mammography, ultrasound, and MRI [abstract]. Radiology 2001; 221(P):230.

[32] Boetes C, Mus RDM, Holland R, et al. Breast tumors: comparative accuracy of MR imaging relative to mammography and US for demonstrating extent. Radiology 1995;197:743–7.

[33] Hlawatsch A, Teifke A, Schmidt M, et al. Preoperative assessment of breast cancer: sonography versus MR imaging. AJR 2002;179: 1493–501.

[34] Kolb TM, Lichy J, Newhouse JH. The impact of bilateral whole breast ultrasound in women with dense breasts and recently diagnosed breast cancer [abstract]. Radiology 2000;217(P): 318.

[35] Berg WA, Gutierrez L, NessAiver MS, et al. Diagnostic accuracy of mammography, clinical examination, US, and MR imaging in preoperative assessment of breast cancer. Radiology 2004; 233:830–49.

[36] Kuhl CK, Schmutzler RK, Leutner CC, et al. Breast MR imaging screening in 192 women proved or suspected to be carriers of a breast cancer susceptibility gene: preliminary results. Radiology 2000;215:267–79.

[37] Warner E, Plewes DB, Hill KA, et al. Surveillance of BRCA1 and BRCA2 mutation carriers with magnetic resonance imaging, ultrasound, mammography, and clinical breast examination. JAMA 2004;292:1317–25.

[38] Warner E, Plewes DB, Shumak RS, et al. Comparison of breast magnetic resonance imaging, mammography, and ultrasound for surveillance of women at high risk for hereditary breast cancer. J Clin Oncol 2001;19:3524–31.

[39] Berg WA. Rationale for a trial of screening breast ultrasound: American College of Radiology Imaging Network (ACRIN) 6666. AJR 2003;180: 1225–8.

[40] Rosen PP. Invasive lobular carcinoma. Rosen's breast pathology. Philadelphia: Lippincott-Raven; 1997. p. 545–65.

[41] Qayyum A, Birdwell RL, Daniel BL, et al. MR imaging features of infiltrating lobular carcinoma of the breast: histopathologic correlation. AJR 2002; 178:1227–32.

[42] Quan ML, Sclafani L, Heerdt AS, et al. Magnetic resonance imaging detects unsuspected disease in patients with invasive lobular cancer. Ann Surg Oncol 2003;10:1048–53.

[43] Rodenko GN, Harms SE, Pruneda JM, et al. MR imaging in the management before surgery of lobular carcinoma of the breast: correlation with pathology. AJR 1996;167:1415–9.

[44] Weinstein SP, Orel SG, Heller R, et al. MR imaging of the breast in patients with invasive lobular carcinoma. AJR 2001;176:399–406.

[45] Yeh ED, Slanetz PJ, Edmister WB, et al. Invasive lobular carcinoma: spectrum of enhancement and morphology on magnetic resonance imaging. Breast J 2003;9:13–8.

[46] Obuchowski NA. Multivariate statistical methods. AJR 2005;185:299–309.

[47] Zurrida S, Costa A, Luini A, et al. The Veronesi quadractomety: an established procedure for the conservative treatment of early breast cancer. J Surg Invest 2001;2:423–31.

[48] Harris RP, Helfand M, Woolf SH, et al. Current methods of the US Preventive Services Task Force: a review of the process. Available at: http://www.ahrq.gov/clinic/ajpmsuppl/harris3. htm. Accessed July 1 2005.

[49] LaTrenta LR, Menell JH, Morris EA, et al. Breast lesions detected with MR imaging: utility and histopathologic importance of identification with US. Radiology 2003;227:856–61.

[50] Liberman L, Bracero N, Morris EA, et al. MRI-guided 9-gauge vacuum-assisted biopsy: initial clinical experience. AJR 2005;185:183–93.

[51] Liberman L, Morris EA, Dershaw DD, et al. Fast MRI-guided vacuum-assisted breast biopsy: initial experience. AJR 2003;181:1283–93.

[52] Morris EA, Liberman L, Dershaw DD, et al. Preoperative MR imaging-guided needle localization of breast lesions. AJR 2002;178:1211–20.

[53] Bartella L, Morris EA, Dershaw DD, et al. Proton MR Spectroscopy (MRS) using choline signal as malignancy marker improves specificity compared to conventional MRI in diagnosis of breast cancer: a preliminary study [abstract]. In: Radiological Society of North America scientific assembly and meeting program, 503. Oak Brook, IL: Radiological Society of North America; 2004.

[54] Lenkinski RE, Katz-Brull R. Breast magnetic resonance spectroscopy. In: Morris EA, Liberman L, editors. Breast MRI: diagnosis and intervention. New York: Springer, Inc.; 2005. p. 266–72.

MAGNETIC RESONANCE IMAGING CLINICS

Magn Reson Imaging Clin N Am 14 (2006) 351–362

Preoperative MR Imaging in Patients with Breast Cancer: Preoperative Staging, Effects on Recurrence Rates, and Outcome Analysis

Uwe Fischer, MD*, Friedemann Baum, MD,
Susanne Luftner-Nagel, MD

- Preoperative questions
- Index tumor size
- Adjacent tissue involvement, extensive intraductal component, multifocality
- Multicentricity
- Involvement of skin, pectoral muscle, or chest wall
- Contralateral breast
- Lymph node status
- Hematogeneous metastases
- False-positive findings on preoperative breast MR imaging
- False-negative findings on preoperative breast MR imaging
- MR imaging after percutaneous biopsy (core biopsy, vacuum biopsy)
- MR imaging early after breast-conserving therapy
- Alteration of primarily planned therapeutic approach
- Influence of MR imaging on recurrence rate and contralateral breast cancer after breast-conserving therapy
- Summary
- References

In industrialized countries, breast cancer is the most common malignant tumor in women. Approximately 10% of all women will suffer from a carcinoma of the breast, and the incidence is increasing. The most important factor affecting survival from this disease is still its early detection at a low stage. Tumors in the intraductal stage or that are less than 1 cm in diameter are especially associated with a greater survival rate. In screening for breast cancer, mammography is the imaging modality of choice. In women with heterogeneously dense or extremely dense breast parenchymal pattern, such as type American College of Radiology (ACR) III or IV; however, the sensitivity

of mammography decreases to 40% to 70%. For this reason, ultrasound scan of the breast has long been recommended as a complementary diagnostic procedure for these women. In recent years, contrast-enhanced MR imaging of the breast has been evaluated increasingly as a complementary method used in combination with mammography. Several studies have found that MR imaging of the breast has the highest sensitivity of all imaging modalities in the detection of invasive breast cancer, especially in dense breasts. This is owing to the depiction of pathologically increased tumor vascularization. Taking all types of breast cancer into account—intraductal as well as invasive—the

Women's Health Care Center, Diagnostisches Brustzentrum Göttingen, Bahnhofsallee 1d 37081, Göttingen, Germany
* Corresponding author.
E-mail address: uwe.fischer-weende@t-online.de (U. Fischer).

combination of mammography with MR imaging has been shown to have the highest sensitivity in the detection of breast cancer. This fact has led to the development of a diagnostic concept, the so-called "OPTIPACK." OPTIPACK is the performance of a dose-reduced one-view digital mammography (MLO-view) in combination with a contrast-enhanced MR imaging of the breast for the early diagnosis of breast carcinoma in the screening situation. Mammography depicts suspicious microcalcifications with high sensitivity and, especially when mammographic interpretation is limited owing to dense parenchymal tissue, MR imaging can depict even small breast tumors with high reliability owing to their increased vascularity. This concept is the most effective in the early detection of breast cancer at the lowest possible radiation dose level. It is, however, also the most expensive concept when compared with established protocols. As well documented for other diseases (ie, lymphoma), an accurate pretherapeutic assessment of the extent of disease is essential for planning the appropriate treatment to get the best long-term results, decrease recurrence rates, and increase patient survival. This article presents an overview of the effects of preoperative local staging with MR imaging in breast cancer patients.

Preoperative questions

The complete excision of all malignant foci is usually the method of choice in the primary treatment of breast cancer. In special constellations, neoadjuvant chemotherapy can precede surgery. Other options such as cryotherapeutic interventions or focused high-energy ultrasound scans are not yet established and are still works-in-progress. Before primary surgical treatment of breast cancer is performed, there are relevant questions that must be answered by the clinical examination and imaging techniques (Figs. 1–3). These questions deal with:

- the precise size of the index tumor
- associated adjacent malignancy (extensive intraductal component [EIC], multifocality)
- multicentricity
- tumor involvement of the skin, pectoral muscle, or chest wall
- contralateral breast
- locoregional lymph node involvement
- hematogeneous metastases (bone, lung, liver, other localizations)

Index tumor size

MR imaging of the breast has been shown to be the most precise imaging modality for the preoperative quantification of the tumor size. In an early study of

Boetes and coworkers [1], no significant difference was found between the size of 61 tumors in preoperative MR imaging measurements and pathologic evaluation. Tumor size was, however, significantly underestimated in 14% of these cases by mammography, and in 18% by ultrasound scan. These results were confirmed by the data of Davis and McCarty [2], as well as of Schelfout and coauthors [3]. In a study by Esserman and coworkers [4], the anatomic extent of breast cancers in 57 patients with 58 carcinomas was accurately predicted more often in preoperative MR imaging examinations than by mammography (MR imaging, 98%; mammography, 55%). In 1996, Rodenko and colleagues [5] had already shown the advantage of MR imaging compared with mammography in the determination of tumor size for the lobular type of breast cancer. In the evaluation of the presented results regarding MR imaging tumor measurements, it must be stated that the histopathologic measurement of the tumor specimen is the gold standard in defining the precise tumor stage.

Adjacent tissue involvement, extensive intraductal component, multifocality

Preoperative information about tumor extension and manifestations in the tissues adjacent to the index tumor is relevant for treatment planning. Depending on the findings, an extended surgical approach may be necessary. The presence of an EIC or additional multifocal tumor manifestations, for example, usually leads to a wider excision (ie, segmental resection or quadrantectomy instead of a tumorectomy or lumpectomy). In this context, multifocality is usually defined as the presence of multiple sites of cancer within one quadrant of the breast. Other definitions specify the distance between the tumor foci (multifocality: less than 3 to 5 cm). Van Goethem and coauthors [6] evaluated the correlation between MR imaging findings and histopathology in patients who have breast cancer showing long spicules or a ductal enhancement pattern near the periphery of the index tumor. In addition, there were some cases of multiple hypervascularized nodules adjacent to the primary carcinoma on MR imaging. In correspondence to these findings, histology findings showed in situ as well as invasive carcinoma in 112 of 128 (87%) cases [6]. Mumtaz and coworkers [7] reported a sensitivity of MR imaging in depicting multifocality and EIC of 81%. Mammography found a respective sensitivity of 62% [7]. In a large study of 177 malignant foci (of which 50% were palpable) in 121 cancerous breasts, Berg and colleagues [8] compared clinical examination and all established imaging modalities

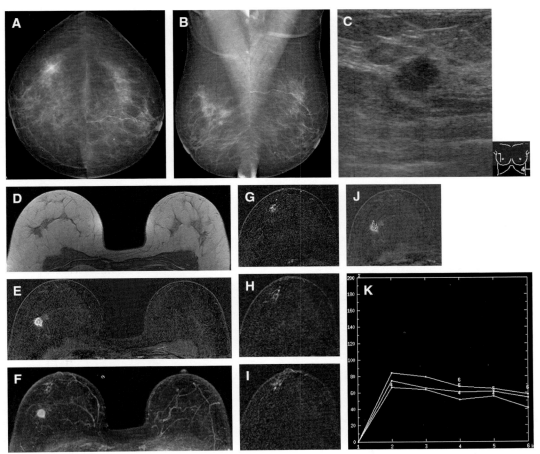

Fig. 1. These images show the digital mammography of both breasts, (*A*) CC view and (*B*) mLO view, of a 69-year-old woman with a palpable mass in the upper outer quadrant of the right breast. Mammograms show an irregularly configured lesion corresponding to the palpable mass (BIRADS category: right breast 4, left breast 1). (*C*) Ultrasound scan shows a round, ill-defined hypoechoic lesion corresponding to the palpable mass in the outer upper quadrant of the right breast (US-BIRADS 4). CE MR mammography shows an ill-defined round lesion on T_1 precontrast image (*D*) with strong peripheral enhancement (rim sign) and white internal septations (*E*). Moreover, maximum intensity projection (MIP) shows an additional dendritic enhancement between the index lesion and the nipple (*F*) (MRM-BIRADS category: right breast 5, left breast 1). (*G,H,I*) Consecutive subtraction images (2nd measurement after contrast administration minus precontrast images) show segmental dendritic enhancement close to the nipple of the breast. (*J,K*) Representative regions-of-interest within the index lesion with moderate initial signal increase and severe wash-out (6 points according to the Goettingen MRM score, MRM-BIRADS 5). Histology after segmentectomy: invasive ductal carcinoma of the right breast pT1c + extensive intraductal component (high grade type), Grading 2, pN0.

separately, as well as in combination. In 19 cases of index tumor and additional EIC, disease extent was underestimated in 39% by mammography, in 37% by ultrasonography, and in only 5% by MR imaging. As expected, the typical MR imaging findings correlating to an EIC were linear, branched clumped enhancement patterns in the tissues adjacent to the index tumor. Corresponding to the detection of EIC, MR imaging was also superior to all other modalities in the depiction of pure intraductal breast cancer (DCIS). The rate of true-

positive findings was 55% for mammography, 47% for ultrasonography, and 89% for MR imaging in this study [8]. Additional multifocal tumor manifestations in 170 patients who had breast cancer were depicted by MR imaging and mammography in 96%, that is, 37% of cases, respectively [3]. The rate of additionally seen multifocal tumor manifestations by MR imaging was 23% in the study performed by Liberman and coworkers [9]. Ikeda and coauthors [10] assessed the value of MR imaging in 59 patients who had EIC. The sensitivity,

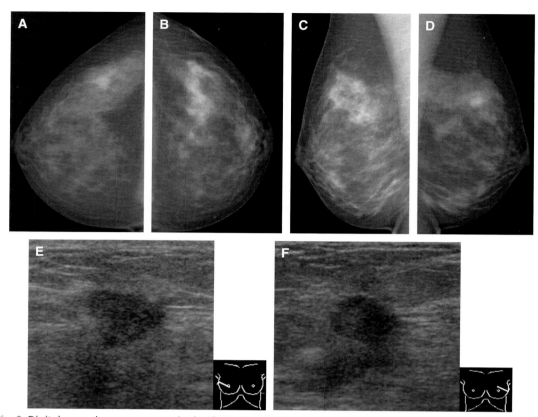

Fig. 2. Digital screening mammography (*A,B*) CC view (*C,D*) mLO view, of both breasts of a 48-year-old woman. There is an ill-defined round lesion seen on both sides in the outer upper quadrant (BIRADS category: right breast 4, left breast 4). (*E,F*) Ultrasound scan shows an ill-defined round lesion with interruption of ligamentous structures corresponding to the suspicious findings on mammogram of both breasts (US-BIRADS category: right breast 5, left breast 5). CE MR mammography shows a hypervascularized round lesion with a ring enhancement in the upper outer quadrant of the right (*G*) and of the left breast (*H*). Additionally, MR imaging depicts another small hypervascularized lesion with a ring enhancement between the lower quadrants of the right breast (*I*). All lesions show washout phenomenon in signal-to-time analysis. (MRM-BIRADS category: right breast 5 [multicentric], left breast 5). (*J*) MR-guided vacuum core biopsy of the lesion between the lower quadrants of the right breast with correctly placed needle equipment. Histology after mastectomy of the right breast and tumorectomy of the left breast: right breast: multicentric invasive carcinomas IDC (12 mm) and ILC (7 mm) pT1c pN0; left breast: invasive ductal carcinoma IDC (8mm) pT1b pN0 CASE 03.

specificity, and accuracy of MR imaging in detecting EIC were 71%, 85%, and 76%, respectively. EIC was characterized by spotty or linear, continuous enhancement from the main tumor to the nipple and by segmental enhancement surrounding the index tumor [10].

Multicentricity

Multicentricity in patients who have breast cancer is one of the most relevant aspects in therapy planning. When multicentricity is proven, mastectomy is recommended instead of breast-conserving therapy. Among the different definitions of multicentricity, the presence of cancer manifestations in more than

one quadrant is the most commonly used definition. Other definitions specify the distance between the tumor foci (multicentricity, more than 3 to 5 cm). In a large study of 170 patients who had breast cancer, MR imaging was reported to depict 95% of the multicentric tumor manifestations. Only 15% of the multicentric tumor manifestations were depicted by mammography [3]. In 70 consecutive women with unilateral breast cancer proven by percutaneous biopsy, Liberman and coauthors [9] reported that MR imaging depicted additional multicentric carcinoma in 7%. Additional sites of cancer were found to be more likely in women with a family history of breast cancer and in patients with infiltrating lobular cancers [9].

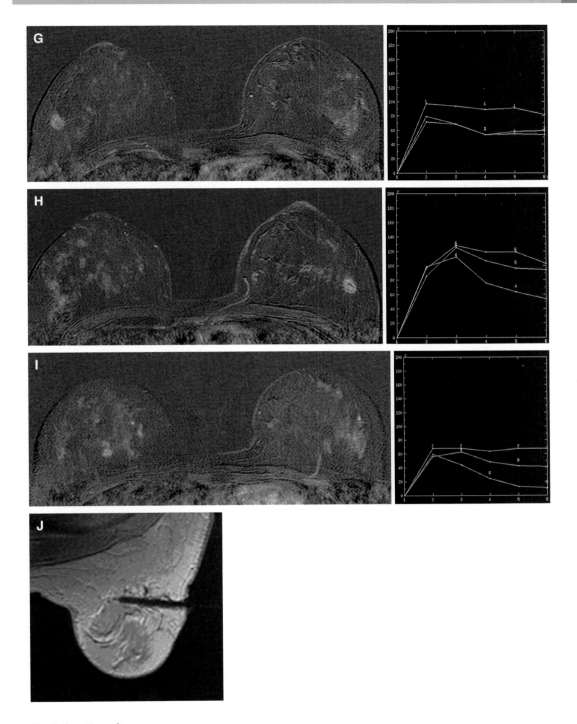

Fig. 2 (*continued*)

Involvement of skin, pectoral muscle, or chest wall

A breast carcinoma with infiltration of cutaneous structures, the pectoral muscle, or the chest wall is classified as a T4-stage tumor. The therapy of such tumors may require a specific approach (ie, preoperative chemotherapy, partial resection of muscle, or chest wall resection). The evaluation of the posterior part of the breast is sometimes

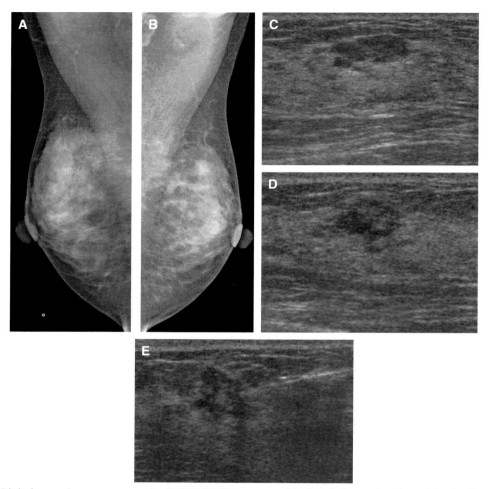

Fig. 3. Digital screening mammography (OPTRIUPACK- concept with digital dose-reduced mLO) (*A,B*). There is an extremely dense parenchym type 4 according to ACR with a possibly round lesion in the upper part of the left breast. There were no calcifications (BIRADS category: right breast 1, left breast 3). Ultrasound scan of the right depicts an oval lesion with well-defined borders and no signs of malignancy in the outer upper quadrant of the left breast (*C*) and an ill-defined hypoechoic lesion nearby (*D*) (BIRADS category: right breast 1 [no image], left breast 3). (*E*) Documentation of the correct placement of the needle during ultrasound-guided core biopsy. CE MR imaging of the breast shows two hypointense lesions in the left breast on precontrast image (*F*). The lesion closer to the skin has high water content on T_2 image, the second lesion nearby shows intermediate signal on T_2 image (*G*). Subtraction image shows hypervascularization of both lesions: the ventral lesion with strong uptake of the contrast material and changes compatible with endotumoral septations, the dorsal lesion with ring enhancement (*H*). Moreover, MR imaging depicts linear enhancement laterally from the described hypervascularized lesions suspicious for additionally intraductal tumor component (*I*). (*J*) Photo documentation of the situation after MR-guided needle localization with positioning of two MR-compatible hook wires (wire 01, wire 02). Situation after injection of the nuclid for sentinel node localization (see hematoma and stripes). Histology after segmentectomy of the left breast: invasive ductal carcinoma IDC + extensive intraductal component pT1b + EIC, pN0. Fibroadenoma.

insufficient in clinical examination, mammography, and even ultrasound scan of larger breasts. MR imaging is superior to these imaging modalities in assessing the possible tumor involvement of the pectoral muscle or the chest wall. Morris and coworkers [11] showed this in 19 patients with posteriorly located breast cancer. Five of these patients (26%) had muscle infiltration at surgery, preoperatively seen only on MR imaging. MR imaging features suggesting such involvement were an obliteration of the retroglandular fat plane and muscle enhancement [11].

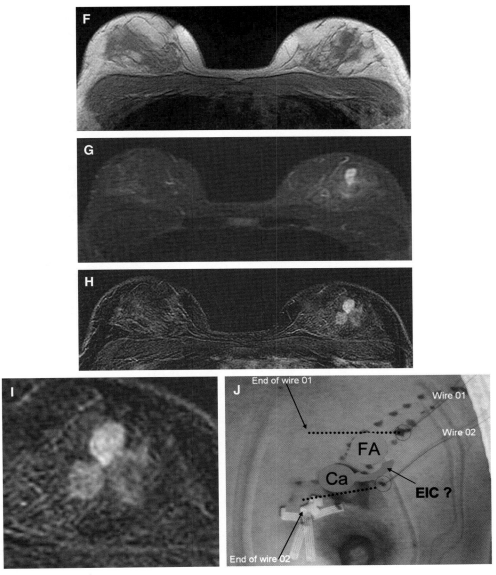

Fig. 3 (*continued*)

Contralateral breast

Patients with breast cancer have an increased risk for carcinoma in the contralateral breast. The rate of synchronous bilateral breast cancer is approximately 3% to 10%. In the above reported study by Berg and coauthors [8], the rate of synchronous bilateral cancer was 9% (10 of 111). Four of the 10 contralateral carcinomas were missed by mammography. Ultrasonography and MR imaging together depicted eight of the contralateral tumor manifestations [8]. The rate of contralateral malignant findings seen only on MR imaging was 6% in an early study of Fischer and coworkers [12,13] and 4% in a follow-up study with an independent patient collective some years later. These data support the results of Liberman and colleagues [14]. They found contralateral breast cancer in 5% of women with breast cancer who underwent contralateral breast MR imaging [14]. In another small collective of patients with breast cancer, MR imaging depicted unexpected contralateral carcinomas in 3 of 34 (8%) cases [15]. In a small study group with a high rate of five synchronous contralateral carcinomas in 17 patients, four of these tumors (24%) were seen on MR imaging alone [16]. The performance of MR imaging of the contralateral breast in addition to conventional imaging techniques after breast-conserving therapy has been shown to increase sensitivity in the detection of breast cancer from 64% to 91%, as well as increase specificity from 84% to 90% [17].

Lymph node status

The lymph node status is the most important known prognostic factor for patients with carcinoma of the breast. For this reason, patients with an invasive carcinoma of the breast usually undergo ipsilateral axillary lymph node dissection. When there are no contraindications, the sentinel node technique is being increasingly performed to reduce morbidity associated with a complete axillary dissection. Patients with DCIS may forgo the axillary dissection. The decision of whether to perform an axillary dissection is dependant on the histopathologically proven tumor stage and cannot be based solely on information gained from imaging techniques. Kvistad and coworkers [18] studied a group of 65 patients who had invasive breast cancer, underwent complete axillary dissection, and were preoperatively evaluated by MR imaging. Using only the signal increase (>100%) as a threshold criterion, the sensitivity of MR imaging was 83% (specificity 90%, accuracy 88%). These results were not improved when lymph node size and morphology were also taken into consideration [18]. Equivalent results were found in a small group of 18 patients using ultrasmall superparamagnetic iron oxide as the contrast material. In this group, the sensitivity for the detection of lymph node metastases was 83% (specificity 96%) [19]. Similar results had already been reported by Mumtaz and coauthors [7] (sensitivity 90%, specificity 82%) and Rodenko and coauthors [5] several years earlier. Although the presented data suggest that MR imaging might be useful in evaluating the lymph node status of breast cancer patients preoperatively, this method has no current relevance for locoregional lymph node staging in these patients.

Hematogeneous metastases

The most common sites of hematogeneous metastatic spread of invasive breast carcinoma are the skeletal system, liver, and lung. Metastases in other organs are more rarely seen. Pretherapeutic staging in patients with breast cancer, therefore, usually includes imaging of the lung (x-ray or spiral computed tomography [sCT]) and the liver (ultrasonography, CT, magnetic resonance tomography [MRT]), as well as a bone scintigraphy. If these techniques show any findings suspicious of metastases,

additional imaging or interventions are performed to complete the diagnostic workup.

False-positive findings on preoperative breast MR imaging

Early studies on the value of preoperative contrast-enhanced MR imaging examinations of the breast criticized the low specificity as a relevant disadvantage of this highly sensitive method. First reports dealing with threshold criteria for the evaluation of breast lesions reported a specificity of approximately 30% to 40% [20]. Since the introduction of multimodal evaluation protocols, which take different morphologic as well as dynamic criteria into consideration, however, the specificity of contrast-enhanced (CE) MRI in subtraction technique has increased and ranges between 75% and 92% [21,22]. This great increase in specificity has resulted in a significant reduction of false-positive findings in preoperatively performed MR imaging studies, as a comparison of the results of MR imaging studies performed at different stages during the development of modern MR imaging protocols verifies [20,23]. In an early small study by Fischer and coworkers [12] in 1994, the rate of false-positive findings in MR imaging performed preoperatively was 5% (4 of 76). A later nonoverlapping study showing a false-positive rate of 4% (16 of 405) supported these earlier results [23]. Recently, other investigators have reported higher rates of false-positive findings. Van Gothem and colleagues [24] reported false-positive findings in 23% of preoperatively performed MR imaging examinations in a study of 67 patients with dense breasts and malignant breast tumors who were to receive breast-conserving surgery. These data correlate with the study results of Liberman and coworkers [9] who reported that additionally detected lesions on MR imaging were benign in 24% of women. Currently there are some working groups with increasing experience in performing MR-guided vacuum biopsies [25–27]. This intervention technique allows a reliable and representative histopathologic assessment of additional suspicious lesions found on preoperative MR imaging. As a consequence, the number of unnecessary open biopsies or widenings of the planned surgical intervention owing to additional MR findings can be reduced.

False-negative findings on preoperative breast MR imaging

The sensitivity of MR imaging in the detection of breast cancer can be evaluated reliably in preoperative MR imaging examinations because most of these patients have a highly suspicious breast lesion or histopathologically verified malignant tumor (index tumor). There are a number of reports dealing with the evaluation of missed carcinoma on MR imaging. Wurdinger and coauthors [28] reported on their analysis of false-negative findings in MR imaging performed preoperatively in 223 patients with 234 histopathologically proven malignant breast lesions (invasive 193, intraductal 41). In this study, the rate of missed carcinoma was reported to be 11.5%, of which 6.4% were invasive and 5.1% intraductal carcinomas. An analysis of the missed breast cancers in MR imaging showed that there was delayed or no contrast enhancement in 4.3%. The missed invasive cancers belonged to the lobular or tubular histologic types. In 7.2% of cases, the carcinoma was not visualized owing to a technical or methodical failure (metal artifacts, lesion outside the field-of-view, incorrect contrast material [CM] injection, motion artifacts, previous core biopsy), or reading errors. A lower rate of false-negative findings on MR imaging was reported by Berg and coauthors [8], who missed 10 of 177 malignant foci (5.6%) on MR mammography. Here also, missed cancers showed low or no CM enhancement. In this study, however, different types of MR imaging systems were used. Sensitivity decreased from 98% when 1.5T systems were used to 92.3% for 1.0T systems. In this context it must be noted that 90% of the missed malignant tumors were examined with 1.0T systems. The results of false-negative MR imaging findings did not negate the indication for surgery made on the grounds of previous mammography or ultrasound findings in this study. All patients underwent histologic evaluation, and no mammographic or sonographic suspicious finding was ignored owing to a normal MR image. However, this study included 424 patients with 488 histopathologically proven lesions (benign and malignant), and 174 of the remaining 254 (68,5%) benign lesions were correctly described as benign on MR imaging [8].

MR imaging after percutaneous biopsy (core biopsy, vacuum biopsy)

Core biopsy or vacuum biopsy is recommended for histopathologic evaluation of suspicious findings in the BI-RADS 4 and 5 categories. This procedure allows a significant reduction of unnecessary open biopsies in patients with benign lesions as well as better pre- and perioperative planning in patients with malignant tumors. But what about MR imaging after previous percutaneous intervention? For core biopsy it has been proven that no disturbing signal changes on postinterventional MR imaging result [29]. In the case of vacuum biopsy, there are no actual data. The relevant information obtained by MR imaging preoperatively, however,

is not the description and demonstration of the index tumor but information about the tumor extent within the other quadrants of the ipsilateral breast as well as a possible synchronous contralateral tumor. With this in mind, it is not likely that previous core or vacuum biopsy decreases the value of preoperative MR imaging. The positioning of a marker after vacuum biopsy also only causes a small susceptibility artifact of a few millimeters when using a coil made of a titanium and nickel alloy. In spite of this, percutaneous interventions should be performed after MR imaging of the breast when possible. This is usually the case if the complete range of diagnostic modalities are in one hand, such as in a diagnostic health care center.

MR imaging early after breast-conserving therapy

To date, there is only one report dealing with the performance of MR mammography soon after breast-conserving therapy and after radiation therapy in 72 patients without preoperative MR mammography. The detection and characterization of depicted lesions was feasible with comparable accuracy in irradiated as well as in nonirradiated breasts [30]. These findings suggest that postoperative "MR staging" of patients who have breast cancer is possible within the first months after starting therapy. It is recommendable, however, to perform MR imaging preoperatively. In our own experience, early postoperative MR imaging with the intent of determining the exact localization and extent of remaining carcinoma tissue in relation to the resection borders in patients with incomplete resection of breast carcinoma (R1-resection) should be avoided.

Alteration of primarily planned therapeutic approach

An upstaging in the preoperative situation may lead to a change in surgical management; however, in some constellations it does not. An extended excision (ie, quandrantectomy or mastectomy instead of a planned lumpectomy) or an additional separate excision (ie, contralateral biopsy) are the typical changes in surgical approach that may be indicated when additional tumor manifestations are found on preoperative imaging. The largest reported patient study with preoperative MR imaging for local staging was performed by Fischer and coworkers [23] in 1999. In a group of 463 patients with a total of 143 histopathologically proven benign lesions and 405 pathologically verified carcinomas, the therapeutic approach was changed correctly in 14.3% owing to the additional information obtained by additional MR mammography. Patients who had findings categorized as BI-RADS 4 and 5 as well as patients with findings of the category BI-RADS 3 were evaluated in this study [23]. In a selected subgroup of these patients with 91 histologically confirmed breast carcinomas, 14% had a primary mastectomy performed instead of the primarily planned breast-conserving therapy owing to the results of the preoperative MR imaging [31]. Bedrosian and colleagues [32] reported the results of preoperative MR imaging in 267 patients who had breast cancer. The planned primary surgical therapy was changed as a consequence of MR imaging results in 20% of the patients. It was shown in a univariate analysis that the change of management was associated significantly with histology. MR imaging gave relevant additional information in 46% of lobular tumors and 24% of ductal carcinomas [32]. In 2004, Schelfout and coauthors [3] published a study of 204 consecutive women with suspicious breast lesions who underwent preoperative MR imaging for staging. Malignant tumors were histologically verified in 170 cases, and the therapeutic approach was correctly changed in 30.6% as a consequence of the MR imaging results. Similar results were reported by Bagley [33], who evaluated a small group of 27 patients with a total of 35 invasive breast cancers and prebiopsy, that is, preoperative MR mammography. In this study, the surgical management was changed in 48% of cases owing to the results of the additional MR imaging.

Influence of MR imaging on recurrence rate and contralateral breast cancer after breast-conserving therapy

The recurrence rate after breast-conserving therapy is reported to be approximately 1% per year after treatment. It can therefore be estimated that there is an average relapse rate of about 5% within the first 5 years after breast-conserving therapy. There is only one recent retrospective study dealing with the outcome of patients with breast cancer in dependence on preoperative local MR staging. Fischer and coworkers [13] studied the benefit of preoperative MR mammography for patients who had breast cancer in comparison with a control group that did not undergo preoperative MR imaging. Preoperative MR imaging was performed in 121 patients (group A). A total of 225 patients had no MR mammography before open biopsy (group B). All patients had histologically proven breast carcinoma. The average follow-up time was 40 respective 41 months. The minimum follow-up was 20 months. Both groups received a comparable established treatment. The performance of a preoperative MR examination reduced the rate of in-breast tumor recurrence from 6.5% (9 of 138) in group B to 1.2% (12 of 35) in group A. Contralateral carcinomas were detected during follow-up in 1.7% (2 of 121) in group A and 4% (9 of 225) in group B. All results were statistically significant ($P < .001$) [13]. These results suggest that *in-breast-recurrence* is not always the correct term to describe the relapse of tumor in the vicinity of the removed index tumors in patients with breast cancer. It is most likely that these "recurrences" correlate with a cancer manifestation that was already existent at the time of the primary diagnosis and treatment of the index tumor. This interpretation is concordant with the experiences of Fisher and colleagues in 1986 [34]. These investigators found that 86% of tumor recurrences within the first 5 years of follow-up were located near the tumor bed or within the same quadrant as the index tumor.

Summary

To assess the individual status of patients with a newly detected breast cancer, the data of all studies show very clearly that the performance of a pretherapeutic local MR staging to detect and evaluate the extent of EIC, multifocality, multicentricity, or synchronous contralateral malignant tumor manifestations is relevant, necessary, and indicated. This MR staging is especially recommended in patients with heterogeneously dense or extremely dense breast tissue pattern on mammography (ACR type III and IV) because the sensitivity of mammography is reduced to 40% to 70% in these patients [8,12,35,36]. Moreover, the presented data suggest that preoperative MR staging is especially important in all cases of histologically verified lobular type of breast cancer. Data from Fischer and colleagues [23] show that preoperative local MR staging can decrease the rate of in-breast tumor relapse as well as the number of metachronous contralateral breast cancers within the follow-up period. These reductions correlate with a better prognosis and a better patient outcome [37,38]. The results of preoperative MR staging are, however, dependent on the adherence to excellent MR technical and methodic standards based on the recommended protocols and respecting aspects of quality assurance. Moreover, there should be the option to perform MR-guided interventions to deal with suspicious findings seen on the additional MR image alone. As a minimum requirement, adequate equipment and proper expertise is necessary to allow for MR-guided preoperative localizations of such lesions. At an optimum, MR image–guided vacuum biopsy allows the minimally invasive histopathologic assessment of unclear enhancing lesions and a reduction of unnecessary additional open biopsies or widening of the primary planned excision. The effective cooperation among the involved radiologists, pathologists, and surgeons must be guaranteed for the optimal management of patient care.

Regarding the cost aspects, MR imaging is the most expensive imaging modality in the diagnostic workup of breast cancer patients. Currently there are no reliable estimations on what the cost effectiveness that a decrease in the tumor recurrence rate or the rate of metachronous contralateral carcinoma in patients with breast cancer who underwent local MR staging would be. Aside from monetary considerations, however, psychological aspects should also be taken into account when decisions on patient management are made.

References

[1] Boetes C, Mus RDM, Holland R, et al. Breast tumors: comparative Accuracy of MR imaging relative to mammography and US for demonstrating extent. Radiology 1995;197:743–7.

[2] Davis PL, McCarty KS. Magnetic resonance imaging in breast cancer staging. Top Magn Reson Imaging 1998;9:60–75.

[3] Schelfout K, van Goethem M, Kersschot E, et al. Contrast-enhanced MR imaging of breast lesions and effect on treatment. Eur J Surg Oncol 2004; 30(5):501–7.

[4] Esserman L, Hylton N, Yassa L, et al. Utility of magnetic resonance imaging in the management of breast cancer: evidence for improved preoperative staging. J Clin Oncol 1999;17(1):110–9.

[5] Rodenko GN, Harms SE, Pruneda JM, et al. MR imaging in the management before surgery of lobular carcinoma of the breast: correlation with pathology. AJR Am J Roentgenol 1996;167(6):1415–9.

[6] van Goethem M, Schelfout K, Kersschot E, et al. Enhancing area surrounding breast carcinoma on MR mammography: comparison with pathological examination. Eur Radiol 2004;14:1363–70.

[7] Mumtaz H, Hall-Craggs MA, Davidson T, et al. Staging of symptomatic primary breast cancer with MR imaging. AJR Am J Roentgenol 1997; 169(2):417–24.

[8] Berg WA, Gutierrez L, NessAiver MS, et al. Diagnostic accuracy of mammography, clinical examination, US, and MR imaging in preoperative assessment of breast cancer. Radiology 2004; 233:830–49.

[9] Liberman L, Morris EA, Dershaw DD, et al. MR imaging of the ipsilateral breast in women with percutaneously proven breast cancer. AJR 2003; 180(4):901–10.

[10] Ikeda O, Nishimura R, Miyayama H, et al. Magnetic resonance evaluation of the presence of an extensive intraductal component in breast cancer. Acta Radiol 2004;45(7):721–5.

[11] Morris EA, Schwartz LH, Drotman MB, et al. Evaluation of pectoralis major muscle in patients with posterior breast tumors on breast MRI: early experiences. Radiology 2000;214:67–72.

[12] Fischer U, Vosshenrich R, Probst A, et al. Preoperative MR mammography in patients with breast cancer – useful help or useless extravagance. RÖFO 1994;161:300–46.

[13] Fischer U, Zachariae O, Baum F, et al. The influence of preoperative MRI of the breasts on recurrence rate in patients with breast cancer. Eur Radiol 2004;14:1725–31.

[14] Liberman L, Morris EA, Kim CM, et al. MR imaging findings of the contralateral breast in women with recently diagnosed breast cancer. AJR 2003; 180(2):333–41.

[15] Rieber A, Merkle E, Bohm W, et al. MRI of histopathologically confirmed mammary carcinoma: clinical relevance of diagnostic procedures for detection of multifocal or contralateral secondary carcinoma. JCAT 1997;21(5):773–9.

[16] Slanetz PJ, Edmister WB, Yeh ED, et al. Occult contralateral breast carcinoma incidentally detected by breast magnetic resonance imaging. Breast J 2002;8(3):145–8.

[17] Viehweg P, Rotter K, Laniado M, et al. MR imaging of the contralateral breast in patients after breast-conserving therapy. Eur Radiol 2004;14:402–8.

[18] Kvistad KA, Rydland J, Smethurst HB, et al. Axillary lymph node metastases in breast cancer: preoperative detection with dynamic contrast-enhanced MRI. Eur Radiol 2000;10(9):1464–7.

[19] Michel SC, Keller TM, Fröhlich JM, et al. Preoperative breast cancer staging: MR imaging of the axilla with ultra-small superparamegnatic iron oxide enhancement. Radiology 2002; 225(2):527–36.

[20] Harms SE, Flaming DP, Hesley KL, et al. MR imaging of the breast with rotating delivery of excitation off resonance: clinical experience with pathological correlation. Radiology 1993;187: 79–84.

[21] Baum F, Fischer U, Vosshenrich R, et al. Classification of hypervascularized lesions in CE MR imaging of the breast. Eur Radiol 2002;12:1087–92.

[22] Kacl GM, Liu P, Debatin, et al. Detection of breast cancer with conventional mammography and contrast-enhanced MR imaging. Eur Radiol 1998;8:194–200.

[23] Fischer U, Kopka L, Grabbe E. Breast carcinoma: effect of preoperative contrast-enhanced MR imaging on the therapeutic approach. Radiology 1999;213(3):881–8.

[24] van Goethem M, Schelfout K, Dijckmans L, et al. MR mammography in the pre-operative staging of breast cancer in patients with dense breast tissue: comparison with mammography and ultrasound. Eur Radiol 2004;14:809–16.

[25] Kuhl CK, Morakkabati N, Leutner CC, et al. MR imaging–guided large-core (14-gauge) needle biopsy of small lesions visible at breast MR imaging alone. Radiology 2001;220:31–9.

[26] Lehman CD, Deperi ER, Peacock S, et al. Clinical experience with MRI-guided vacuum-assisted breast biopsy. AJR 2005;184:1782–7.

[27] Liberman L, Bracero N, Morris F, et al. MRI-guided 9-gauge vacuum-assisted breast biopsy: Initial clinical experience. AJR 2005;185:183–93.

[28] Wurdinger S, Kamrath S, Eschrich D, et al. False-negative findings of malignant breast lesions on preoperative magnetic resonance mammography. Breast 2001;10:131–9.

[29] Fischer U, Vosshenrich R, Kopka L, et al. CE dynamic MR mammography after diagnostic and therapeutic interventions of the breast. Bildgebung 1996;63:94–100.

[30] Morakkabati N, Leutner CC, Schmiedel A, et al. Breast MR imaging during or soon after radiation therapy. Radiology 2003;229:893–901.

[31] Gatzemeier W, Liersch T, Stylianou A. Preoperative MR mammography in breast carcinoma. Effect on operative treatment from the surgical viewpoint. Chirurg 1999;70(12):1460–8.

[32] Bedrosian I, Mick R, Orel SG, et al. Changes in the surgical treatment of patients with breast carcinoma based on preoperative magnetic resonance imaging. Cancer 2003;98(3):468–73.

[33] Bagley FH. The role of magnetic resonance imaging mammography in the surgical management of the index breast cancer. Arch Surg 2004;139:380–3.

[34] Fisher ER, Sass R, Fisher B, et al. Pathologic findings from the National Surgical Adjuvant Breast Project (protocol 6). II. Relation of local breast recurrence to multicentricity. Cancer 1986;57:1717–24.

[35] Blümke DA, Gatsonis CA, Chen MH, et al. Magnetic resonance imaging of the breast prior to biopsy. JAMA 2004;292:2735–42.

[36] Hlawatsch A, Teifke A, Schmidt M, et al. Preoperative assessment of breast cancer: sonography versus MR imaging. AJR 2002;179(6):1493–501.

[37] Hölzel D, Engel J, Schmidt M, et al. Modell zur primären und sekundären Metastasierung beim Mammakarzinom und dessen klinischer Bedeutung. Strahlenther Onkol 2001;1:10–4.

[38] Moran MS, Haffty BG. Local-regional breast cancer recurrence: prognostic groups based on pattern of failure. Breast J 2002;8:81–7.

ELSEVIER
SAUNDERS

MAGNETIC
RESONANCE
IMAGING CLINICS

Magn Reson Imaging Clin N Am 14 (2006) 363–378

A Clinical Oncology Perspective on the Use of Breast MR

Monica Morrow, MD[a,b,*], Gary Freedman, MD[c]

- Current outcomes of breast-conserving therapy
  Selection of local therapy
  Local control
  The impact of MR on selection of surgical procedure
- MR for identification of local recurrence after breast-conserving therapy
- Other applications of MR
  Breast-conserving surgery without radiation
  Partial breast irradiation
- Summary
- References

Over the last 30 years, the surgical treatment of breast cancer has evolved from the routine use of radical mastectomy to a patient-driven choice between total mastectomy and breast-conserving surgery with radiation (BCT) for most women with ductal carcinoma in situ (DCIS) and stage one and stage two breast cancer. As BCT has matured from an experimental treatment to an accepted standard of care, important lessons have been learned about patient selection for the procedure, the role of radiotherapy in maintaining local control, and the detection and management of local recurrence. A large database of patient outcomes from both randomized trials and observational studies exists and provides a standard against which the benefits of therapeutic modifications must be measured. The lack of a survival difference between BCT and mastectomy [1–6], is well established. Currently, the selection of local therapy is based on a history, physical examination findings, and diagnostic mammography results [7]. The development

of MR imaging of the breast has raised important questions about how this modality should be integrated into the initial evaluation and posttherapy follow-up of women who have breast cancer. This article considers the current data on patient selection for local therapy; the incidence, detection, and management of local recurrence after BCT; the status of both whole and partial breast irradiation; and the impact of MR on these outcomes. These measures were chosen because they reflect standard oncologic endpoints—disease-free survival and quality of life, which are evaluated when new therapeutic modalities are considered.

Current outcomes of breast-conserving therapy

Selection of local therapy

Standards for the local therapy of invasive carcinoma were published first by a joint committee of the American College of Surgeons, American

a Department of Surgical Oncology, Fox Chase Cancer Center, 333 Cottman Avenue, Suite C302, Philadelphia, PA 19111, USA
b Temple University, 1801 North Broad Street, Philadelphia, PA 19122, USA
c Department of Radiation Oncology, Breast Evaluation Center, Fox Chase Cancer Center, 333 Cottman Avenue, Suite P1074, Philadelphia, PA 19111, USA
* Corresponding author. Department of Surgical Oncology, Fox Chase Cancer Center, 333 Cottman Avenue, Suite C302, Philadelphia, PA 19111.
E-mail address: monica.morrow@fccc.edu (M. Morrow).

1064-9689/06/$ – see front matter © 2006 Elsevier Inc. All rights reserved.
mri.theclinics.com

doi:10.1016/j.mric.2006.07.006

College of Radiology, and College of American Pathologists in 1992 [8] and have been updated regularly [9] and expanded to include DCIS [10]. Absolute contraindications to BCT include a history of prior therapeutic irradiation to the breast region, the inability to obtain negative margins after a reasonable number of surgical attempts, first and second trimester pregnancy, and clinically or mammographically detected multicentric cancer. These contraindications appear to be identified reliably with a history and physical examination and diagnostic mammography [7,11,12]. Morrow and coauthors [7] reported that of 216 consecutive patients thought to be candidates for BCT after clinical evaluation and diagnostic mammography, BCT was performed successfully in 210 (97.2%). Kearney and Morrow [13] also reported that of 90 patients with a positive margin after an initial diagnostic or therapeutic surgical excision who had no apparent clinical or mammographic contraindications to BCT, breast conservation was performed successfully in 96%. Of the 216 patients included in the study of Morrow and coauthors [7], only 14 had infiltrating lobular carcinoma. It has been suggested that in patients with infiltrating lobular carcinoma, the selection of surgical therapy is more problematic than for those with ductal carcinoma [14,15]. Yeatman and coworkers [14] reported that patients with infiltrating lobular carcinoma were 2.5 times more likely to require conversion from lumpectomy to mastectomy than their counterparts with infiltrating ductal carcinoma. However, this conclusion was based on only 73 patients with lobular carcinoma. In a much larger study, Arpino and colleagues [16] compared outcomes in 4140 patients with lobular carcinoma with those of 45,169 patients with infiltrating ductal carcinoma. A slightly higher rate of BCT (12.7%) was seen in the ductal group than in the lobular group (9.5%, *P* = .0001). However, in both the study of Yeatman and coworkers [14] and Arpino and coworkers [16], patients with lobular cancer had significantly larger tumors than those with ductal carcinoma, and no adjustment was made for this difference. In addition, the extremely low rate of BCT in the study of Arpino and coworkers [16] makes it difficult to determine the implications of the small reported difference in the use of BCT in practice today when much higher rates of BCT are seen. To examine issues related to the surgical treatment of lobular carcinoma, Morrow and colleagues [17] compared outcomes of 318 patients with lobular carcinoma (pure or mixed) with those of 636 patients with ductal carcinoma. Each patient who had lobular cancer was compared with two control patients who had ductal cancer matched for year of diagnosis, menopausal status, and pathologic stage. Using

clinical and mammographic evaluation, 33% of patients who had lobular cancer were considered not to be candidates for BCT compared with 28% of those who had ductal carcinoma (odds ratio 1.47, 95% CI 1.02, 2.13) consistent with the mean size of the tumors in the lobular group (2.63 cm) being significantly larger than in the ductal group (2.06 cm, *P* < .001). However, in the remaining women felt to be candidates for BCT, the procedure was equally successful between those with ductal and lobular carcinoma after adjustment for tumor size and patient age. Failure of BCT occurred in 9.7% of the lobular group and 9.3% of the ductal group (*P* = .43) [17]. This observation is consistent with the finding of Arpino and coauthors [16] that in patients felt to be candidates for BCT using standard clinical and imaging evaluation, little difference in the ability to complete the procedure is seen based on tumor histology.

Even when the subset of patients who have tumors of any histology that are palpable but not seen on imaging studies is considered, it is difficult to find evidence that the performance of BCT is problematic. Morrow and coauthors [12] compared 52 patients who had clinically evident but mammographically occult breast cancer with 217 women who had both clinically and mammographically evident tumors treated during the same period. Eligibility for BCT did not differ between groups, with 67% of those with occult tumors felt to be candidates for BCT compared with 70% of those with evident tumors (*P* value not significant). Breast-conserving therapy was performed successfully in an equal proportion of patients who elected to have the procedure in both groups. These findings indicate that for tumors not visualized mammographically, clinical evaluation provides an accurate estimate of the extent of malignancy and the potential success of BCT. The available literature indicates that patients can be reliably selected for BCT using clinical examination and mammography and does not document a major problem in treatment selection for women with lobular carcinoma.

Local control

The goal of BCT is to minimize the incidence of local recurrence while maintaining a good cosmetic outcome. Local recurrence rates in the initial trials comparing BCT with mastectomy are summarized in Table 1 [1–6]. It is noteworthy that although patients were entered into these studies at a time when mammographic techniques were not developed fully, pathologic evaluation of resection margins was limited, and many women with small cancers did not receive adjuvant systemic therapy, the majority of studies did not show significant differences in the incidence of local failure between patients

Table 1: **Local recurrence in trials of BCT versus mastectomy**

			Local recurrence	
Trial	No. of patients	Follow-up (yr)	BCT (%)	Mastectomy
Institut Gustave Roussy [1]	179	15	9	14
Milan I [3]	701	20	9	2
NSABP B06 [2]	1219	20	14	10
NCI [5]	237	18	22	6
EORTC [4]	874	10	20	12
Danish [6]	904	6	3	4

treated with mastectomy and those undergoing lumpectomy to negative margins followed by radiotherapy. The high local failure rates reported in the National Cancer Institute (NCI) study [5] and the European Organisation for Research and Treatment of Cancer (EORTC) study [4] reflect the fact that histologically negative margins were not required for lumpectomy patients in these trials. More recent findings indicate that as increasing experience has been gained with BCT, local recurrence rates have decreased considerably and are routinely less than 10% at 10 years, and in many cases less than 5% [18–26]. Extremely low rates of local failure are observed in multiple settings, not only in institutions with specialized breast practices. In a recent review of National Surgical Adjuvant Breast and Bowel Project (NSABP) trials, Wapnir and colleagues [23] reported that 10-year local failure rates were less than 5% for both estrogen receptor positive and negative patients who received adjuvant systemic therapy in a number of different protocols. The reasons for this are multifactorial and were addressed by Pass and coauthors [27] in a study examining the impact of changes in processes of care on local recurrence rates in a group of 607 patients treated at a single institution between 1981 and 1996. The rate of ipsilateral breast tumor recurrence at 5 years decreased from 8% in patients treated between 1981 and 1985 to 1% for those treated between 1991 and 1996. During this period, the proportion of patients with negative margins increased from 48% to 76%, and the mean number of pathology slides examined to determine margin status increased from 10.6 per patient to 21.1 per patient ($P < .001$). The total radiation dose also increased significantly, with 26% of the patients treated in the earlier period receiving a dose of less than 51 Gray compared with none of the patients in the later period. A significant increase in tamoxifen use, from 10% to 61% of cases, was also noted. In a similar study, Ernst and coworkers [28] observed that 8-year rates of locoregional recurrence after BCT decreased from 20.1% to 5.4% in patients treated between 1985 and 1992 and 1993 and 1999, respectively ($P = .0018$). In contrast, no change in the incidence of locoregional recurrence after mastectomy was observed between the two time periods. This finding emphasizes an important point. There are two mechanisms of local recurrence in the breast after BCT. The first is caused by a microscopic residual tumor burden too large to be controlled by irradiation, and the second is similar to chest wall recurrence after mastectomy in which local recurrence occurs as a first site of metastases [29]. The former mechanism is responsible for the increased rate of local failure seen in patients who have positive margins after lumpectomy. Improvements in imaging, patient selection, evaluation of the adequacy of resection, and definition of an optimal dose of radiotherapy have resulted in a reduction in this type of recurrence as experience with breast-conserving surgery has been gained. The second type of recurrence is more problematic to eliminate. The increased use of systemic therapy for the treatment of small node-negative breast cancers and the development of more effective systemic therapies has resulted in a small decrease in recurrences owing to this mechanism. This thesis is supported by the results of the ATAC (Arimidex, Tamoxifen Alone or in Combination trial) comparing the efficacy of anastrazole to tamoxifen [30]. In this study, anastrazole was found to be superior to tamoxifen in improving disease-free survival (hazard ratio 0.83, 95% CI 0.71-0.96). In addition to reducing the number of distant metastases, anastrazole decreased the number of local failures from 83 to 67, a 20% reduction. However, the stability of local failure rates after mastectomy over time [28] indicates that elimination of this type of recurrence awaits more substantial improvements in adjuvant systemic therapy.

The impact of MR on selection of surgical procedure

The background information discussed above is useful when considering the role of MR in treatment selection for the woman with known carcinoma. BCT is now an established therapy with well-defined selection criteria. Local recurrences owing to improper patient selection or inadequate local therapy are infrequent. Yet, a substantial number of studies have found that the performance of MR in women with localized cancers identifies additional tumor foci in 11% to 31% of cases (Table 2) [31–41]. The demonstration of these additional tumor foci has been used to argue that MR should be a routine part of the preoperative evaluation of women with breast carcinoma.

A smaller number of studies have examined the actual impact of MR findings on surgical therapy. Bedrosian and colleagues [36] reported that surgical management was altered in 69 of 267 patients (26%). The most common change was conversion from breast conservation to mastectomy in 44, with wide excision and biopsy through a separate incision accounting for the other modifications. However, pathologic verification of malignancy occurred in only 71% of these cases. Berg and coauthors [39] observed that MR resulted in wider excision than initially planned in 30% of women undergoing breast-conserving surgery, although disease extent was overestimated in 20 of the 29. In the study of Deurloo and coworkers [40], 15% of patients underwent mastectomy and 67% wider excision based on MR findings. In contrast to studies examining the role of MR in breast cancer patients in general, in which approximately one quarter of patients have additional tumor identified, findings in patients with lobular carcinoma suggest that approximately 50% will have their management altered (Table 3) [42–46]. In the study of Weinstein and colleagues [42], 18 patients with infiltrating lobular carcinoma had MR imaging before surgical excision. In nine of these cases, MR did not add to the information provided by conventional imaging. In two cases, MR identified a palpable primary lesion that was not seen on other imaging modalities, whereas in five cases, additional disease was seen, although its extent was overestimated in one case. In the other 14 patients, MR was performed after an excisional biopsy, and

Table 2: MR imaging of the ipsilateral breast in women with known carcinoma

Study	No. of cancers	Additional tumor (%)
Orel et al [31]	64	20
Boetes et al [32]	61	15
Mumtaz et al [33]	92	11
Fischer et al [34]	336	16
Drew et al [35]	178	23
Bedrosian et al [36]	267	15
Liberman et al [37]	70	27
Bluemke et al [38]	428	13
Berg et al [39]	96	31
Deurloo et al [40]	116	23

Table 3: Studies of MR in patients with lobular carcinoma

Study	No. of cases	Additional cancer (%)
Weinstein et al [42]	32	50
Munot et al [46]	14	50
Kneeshaw et al [43]	21	24
Quan et al [45]	62	61
Schelfout et al [44]	26	34

in nine, findings consistent with residual tumor were noted. However, the margin status of these patients is not provided and in patients with tumor involving the lumpectomy margin, the need for additional surgery is already established. If patients with potentially positive margins and clinically evident, but mammographically occult, lesions are excluded, the potential benefit of MR is reduced to 22% of the study population. Quan and coauthors [45] reported that 38 of 62 (61%) patients with lobular cancer had additional suspicious lesions identified by MR, although only 11 had additional carcinoma documented. The available data suggest that as many as one third to one half of patients with lobular cancer have significant amounts of tumor that is not identified by conventional evaluation [42–46]. This finding suggests that the treatment of lobular cancer with less than mastectomy would be unsuccessful in a significant number of cases. This assumption is not borne out by the available clinical data. As discussed previously, the work of Morrow and coworkers [17] and Arpino et al [16] indicates that patients who have lobular carcinoma can be selected for BCT with the same success rate as those who have ductal carcinoma. Local failure rates for patients who have lobular carcinoma do not differ significantly from those seen in patients who have infiltrating ductal cancer who are treated with BCT. Studies addressing this issue are summarized in Table 4 [20,47–52] and show absolutely no trend toward an increased risk of local failure in patients with lobular carcinoma, even with long-term follow-up. The study of Peiro and colleagues [48] included 1624 patients with a median follow-up of 133 months for survivors. Pathology slides were reviewed in 82% of cases, and 93 patients were found to have pure lobular carcinoma, and an additional 59 had mixed ductal and lobular cancer. Local recurrence rates did not differ on the basis of histology, and in multivariate analysis, histologic type was not a significant predictor of survival or recurrence. Similar findings were reported by Santiago and coauthors [49] in a study with a median follow-up of 8.7 years. The 5-year and 10-year local failure rates were 14% and 18% for patients with

Table 4: **Local failure after breast conservation therapy: lobular versus ductal carcinoma**

Study	No. of lobular cases	LR (%)	
		Lobular	*Ductal*
Smitt et al [20]	49	12	11
Weiss et al [50]	41 pure, 23 mixed	6	6
White et al [51]	30	3.3	4.2
Winchester et al [47]	146		
	Stage I	2	3
	Stage II	5	4
Peiro et al [48]	93 pure	15	13
	59 mixed	13	13
Molland et al [52]	182	3.9	5.3
Santiago et al [49]	55	12	18

Abbreviation: LR, local recurrence.

lobular carcinoma compared with 6% and 12% for invasive ductal carcinoma ($P = .24$). There were also no differences in the rate of contralateral carcinoma on the basis of histology. Both the studies of Santiago and coworkers [49] and the study of Peiro and coworkers [48] were single-institution studies, and the ability to generalize their findings to multiple practice settings could be considered questionable. However, Winchester and coworkers [47] used data from the National Cancer database on 291,273 women who had operable breast cancer treated in a variety of settings across the United States to address this question. For the subset of 1953 patients treated with BCT between 1985 and 1988, no differences in 5-year local disease-free survival between women who had ductal and lobular carcinoma, were noted, supporting the observations from single institution reports with longer follow-up periods.

Tillman and coauthors [53] attempted to assess the net benefit of MR in the evaluation of the breast cancer patient by assessing clinical information and pathology reports as well as imaging findings. The effect of MR was judged to be strongly favorable (8%) or somewhat favorable (3%) in 11% of cases,

somewhat unfavorable (5%) or strongly unfavorable (1%) in 6% of cases, and uncertain in 2%. However, this study, like all of the studies of the impact of MR on choice of surgical procedure, makes the assumption that the identification of additional tumor corresponding to the MR abnormality is proof that the MR was beneficial to the patient. This is an assumption that is open to question and lies at the crux of the debate regarding what evidence of clinical benefit is needed before the adoption of MR into routine clinical practice.

Although clinically multicentric carcinoma is recognized in fewer than 10% of patients [54,11], the multifocal/centric nature of breast cancer has long been recognized by pathologists. Studies using serial subgross sectioning to evaluate clinically and mammographically normal tissue from the breasts of women thought to have localized tumors have found additional tumor foci in 21% to 63% of cases (Table 5) [55–62]. In one such study, [56] a quadrantectomy of the tumor-bearing area of the breast was performed on the mastectomy specimen in 203 patients thought to have localized carcinoma. Residual microscopic carcinoma was found in 33%. The work of Holland and coauthors [62] provided

Table 5: **Pathologic studies of multifocality/multicentricity**

Study	No. of cases	Population	Multifocal/centric (%)
Qualheim and Gall [55]	157	Not stated	54
Rosen et al [56]	203	Invasive carcinoma	33
Lagios [57]	85	Not stated	21
Egan [58]	118	Not stated	60
Schwartz et al [59]	43	Nonpalpable cancer	44
Vaidya et al [60]	30	Invasive carcinoma	63
Anastassiades et al [61]	366	Invasive ≤7 cm, noninvasive	49
Holland et al [62]	282	Clinically unicentric invasive cancer <5 cm	63

detailed information on the distribution and type of residual carcinoma found outside the confines of the grossly identified tumor. Holland and co-workers studied 282 mastectomy specimens from patients with grossly unicentric carcinomas ≤4 cm in size and found that all carcinoma was confined to the site of the primary tumor in only 37% of cases and was within 2 cm in an additional 20%. However, the majority of foci of residual disease were found within 4 cm of the primary site, and the likelihood of identifying residual tumor was not related to the size of the primary tumor. In a subsequent study, Holland and coworkers [63] found that the presence of an extensive intraductal component (EIC) in association with the invasive carcinoma was strongly correlated with the distribution of residual tumor beyond the primary site with 74% of EIC-positive patients having disease outside the primary tumor site compared with 42% of EIC-negative patients ($P = .00001$). The majority of the multicentric tumor foci were intraductal carcinoma. Pathology studies such as these were used to argue strongly that the treatment of breast cancer with less than total mastectomy was inappropriate. However, extensive clinical experience [1–6,18–22] has shown that the majority of these subclinical foci are controlled with radiotherapy. In the NSABP B06 trial [2], the ipsilateral breast tumor recurrence rate was 14% at 20 years in patients receiving radiotherapy (RT), compared with 39% in those who did not receive RT, indicating that these subclinical foci are biologically relevant even if they have little clinical impact on the patient receiving whole-breast irradiation.

It is reasonable to ask whether the additional tumor foci identified by MR are the same tumor foci identified by the pathologist. The available evidence would suggest that they are. Sardanelli and coworkers [64] performed MR on 90 patients who were scheduled to undergo mastectomy. Serial subgross sectioning was performed on the mastectomy specimens, and tumor location was mapped and correlated with the findings of the MR examination. The overall sensitivity of MR was 81%; 89% for invasive foci and 40% for in situ disease. The mean diameter of malignant lesions not seen by MR was 5 mm (range 0.5 to 15.0 mm). In the 90 breasts studied, MR failed to identify microscopic multifocal or multicentric disease in 19 and incorrectly suggested additional foci of malignancy in 30 cases. These findings strongly suggest that MR is capable of detecting some but not all of the tumor foci found with detailed pathologic sectioning. The findings of Berg and colleagues [39] and Liberman and coauthors [37] also support the idea that the same tumor is identified with both techniques. Berg and colleagues [39] observed that in 40 of 46 breasts (87%) with additional tumor foci, the foci were within 4 cm of the index lesion. Liberman and colleagues [37] also noted that the majority of additional tumor foci were in the same quadrant as the index lesion. These patterns correspond well to the pathologic distribution of tumor described by Holland and coauthors [62] in which 96% of tumor foci were within 4 cm of the index tumor.

If the cancer identified by MR is the same cancer that has been treated successfully with radiotherapy for the last 30 years, how does its identification improve clinical management? One study [65] has attempted to address the influence of preoperative MR on local recurrence rates in patients treated with BCT. Fischer and coworkers [65] retrospectively compared the local failure rates in 86 patients who had conventional imaging studies plus an MR before BCT with 138 patients who had only conventional imaging. After a mean follow-up of 40.3 months in the MR group and 41 months in the conventional imaging group, local recurrences were observed in 1.2% and 6.8% of patients, respectively ($P < .001$). Unfortunately, the retrospective nature of the study resulted in some imbalances among the groups, which render the results extremely difficult to interpret. For example, only 5% of patients in the MR group did not receive adjuvant therapy compared with 18% in the conventional imaging group. It is well documented in randomized trials that the use of adjuvant systemic therapy decreases the risk of local failure by approximately 50% [66–68], so this imbalance could be responsible for the difference in the rates of local failure that was observed. Because of these problems, this study cannot be considered evidence of a clinical benefit for MR.

Currently, there is no convincing evidence that the use of MR for patient selection improves local control in women undergoing BCT. It has been suggested that the use of preoperative MR, by allowing better definition of the extent of disease, would decrease the need for re-excision for positive margins [69]. However, in practice, it may be difficult to translate imaging findings to the three-dimensional surgical setting. An initial report of a 43% positive margin rate in 21 patients undergoing MR-guided localization and excision does not provide convincing evidence of the utility of MR to achieve negative margins [70]. In comparison, Staradub and colleagues [71] reported an 80% negative margin rate in 217 patients with nonpalpable cancers when the extent of disease was defined by mammography and ultrasonography. In practice, there are multiple factors that influence margin status including lesion type (calcification or mass), surgeon experience, and philosophy regarding what constitutes an adequate resection of normal breast tissue, all of which influence the rate of negative margins after a single excision. Neither the impact of MR on local recurrence nor its effect on the number of resections needed to obtain negative margins can be assessed without a properly designed, prospective, randomized trial. The performance of such a trial in unselected women undergoing BCT would require an enormous sample size owing to the low rates of local failure that are currently seen. In a recent review of NSABP trials, 10-year rates of local recurrence were less than 5% for patients receiving adjuvant systemic therapy [23]. Given the cost of the MR examination and the additional biopsies generated, it is unlikely that decreases in local failure rates of less than 3% to 5% would be considered meaningful. A trial focusing on a group at higher risk of local failure such as very young women with breast cancer [72–74] would require fewer subjects and would have the advantage of addressing an actual clinical problem. Convincing data indicate that women 45 or younger at diagnosis are at increased risk of local recurrence after BCT, but not after mastectomy, compared with their older counterparts [72–74]. This information suggests that improvements in aspects of local therapy such as patient selection have the potential to decrease local failure rates in the younger age group. Although local recurrence would be the primary study endpoint, the number of surgical excisions to achieve negative margins would be a secondary endpoint for which data would be available in the short term. However, resources for clinical trials are limited, and this would still be a large and expensive study to conduct to determine if local recurrence rates are reduced by a few percent.

MR for identification of local recurrence after breast-conserving therapy

The current recommendations for the detection of local recurrence in the preserved breast are patient self-examination monthly, physician examination every 3 to 6 months for 5 years and then annually, and an initial mammogram 6 to 12 months after radiation and then yearly [9]. As discussed previously, improvements in selection of patients for BCT using clinicopathologic factors and the use of adjuvant systemic therapy, have resulted in 10-year local recurrence rates of less than 5% for patients receiving chemotherapy or tamoxifen [23]. The median interval to local recurrence is approximately 5 to 6 years for patients treated with BCT [26,75–77]. In one study, the median interval was 3.7 years with radiation alone, 5 years with chemotherapy with or without hormonal therapy, and 6.7 years with hormonal therapy alone [18]. Routine use of MR for posttreatment imaging would therefore require patients to

undergo at least yearly scanning for up to 10 years after treatment. In many cases, with 6-month follow-up studies ordered for indeterminate findings or false-positive results, twice-a-year scanning would be performed. Seventy-five percent of the more than 200,000 new breast cancer cases in the United States are early-stage invasive breast cancers, and approximately 70% (140,000 women) are treated with breast-conserving surgery and postoperative radiation [78]. Therefore, the MR capacity needed to begin routine surveillance of all these irradiated women for 10 years or more would be enormous. More importantly, there is no obvious rationale for screening for local recurrence with MR.

Radiation therapy results in fibrosis of the treated breast, but this does not prevent detection of recurrences by physical examination and mammography, and approximately one third to one half of local recurrences are detected by mammography alone [77,79–84]. Evidence suggests that current methods of surveillance for local recurrence are highly successful, with an average recurrence size in the range of 1 to 2 cm [85–89]. Mastectomy is the standard treatment of an isolated local recurrence after BCT, and 85% to 90% of patients have operable disease at the time of detection of the local recurrence [75,81,89–92]. Earlier detection of tumors at a smaller size may not have an impact on salvage treatment that is already highly successful. Salvage mastectomy for local recurrence results in local control rates of approximately 85% to 95% [75,79–81,83,90,92]. The size of a recurrent tumor is not a prognostic factor in most series of patients who have local recurrence after radiation, with the majority of studies identifying invasive recurrence, skin involvement, or initial tumor size and nodal status [75,79,80,84,93,94] as important prognostic factors. Regardless of the size at which the recurrence is identified, further attempts at breast conservation are not considered standard therapy because of the higher risk of further local failure after treatment with excision alone. The incidence of a second local failure after wide excision is 19% to 48%, even with strict selection criteria of tumors less than 2 cm in size, the absence of skin involvement, and negative resection margins [75,83,84,92,95,96].

Finally, the idea that the "earlier" identification of local recurrence with MR will improve outcome does not appear to reflect accurately the biology of local recurrence. Most studies indicate that a shorter time to the development of local recurrence is a negative prognostic factor; an indication of aggressive tumor biology rather than "early detection" as a result of the surveillance intervention. Veronesi and coauthors [89] reported that the risk of distant metastases after a local recurrence occurring within 1 year of initial treatment was 6.6 times the risk seen in patients who have local recurrence more than 3 years after surgery (P = .004). Other studies have confirmed higher rates of distant metastases and worse survival rates with shorter intervals to isolated local recurrence [4,88,93,97–99].

Other applications of MR

Rather than using MR to select patients for BCT, a problem that has been largely solved, a different approach would be to focus on using MR to identify patients who do not require whole-breast radiation therapy. The need for radiation after lumpectomy is a major concern for women and a common reason that women who are medically eligible for BCT choose to undergo mastectomy [78,100]. Below we review the data from trials of whole-breast and partial-breast RT and examine the potential of MR to affect this aspect of treatment.

Breast-conserving surgery without radiation

Although breast-conserving surgery and radiation have resulted in long-term disease control and overall survival rates equal to that seen after mastectomy [2,3], patient concerns about radiation and its time and expense have stimulated interest in determining whether radiation is necessary for all patients. There have been several prospective, randomized trials of breast-conserving surgery with or without radiation therapy for stage I and II breast cancer (Table 6) [2,101–109]. The studies of conservative surgery without tamoxifen found a significant reduction in the risk of local recurrence with the addition of radiation, with local recurrence rates decreasing from 24% to 39% without radiation to 4% to 14% with radiation [2,102,103,106]. In one prospective study of conservative surgery alone in a highly selected favorable patient population consisting of women with T1 tumors, ductal histology, no extensive in situ component, absence of lymphovascular invasion, resection margin ≥1 cm, and negative axillary nodes, the incidence of local recurrence was 23% after a median follow-up of 7.2 years [110,111]. Tamoxifen is not a substitute for radiotherapy [104,105,107]. In the NSABP B21 study, patients receiving tamoxifen only had an 8-year local failure rate of 16.5% compared with 9.3% for those receiving RT only and 2.8% for those treated with RT and tamoxifen [104]. These initial attempts to identify patients in whom radiation may be omitted were based on a gross total resection of the primary tumor with various degrees of pathologic margin assessment and the presence of unifocal disease in the breast after evaluation with combinations of mammography, ultrasonography, and physical examination.

The rationale for postoperative radiation therapy is to treat microscopic residual disease that may exist in the breast after conservative surgery and act a source of local recurrence. In patients undergoing re-excision after an initial excisional biopsy, residual disease near the biopsy cavity is present in 21% to 62% of cases [112–116]. As discussed previously, pathologic studies of mastectomy specimens after local excision of apparently unicentric tumors confirm that there is residual disease in 21% to 63% of patients [57,60,62]. Even after breast-conserving surgery with a 2-cm margin, residual disease is present in 17% to 60% of patients [117,62,63,118]. One potential role of MR would be to identify patients in whom microscopic foci of residual disease was not present, because this subset of patients is least likely to require whole-breast irradiation. Although MR is able to detect some of this residual disease after surgery, available data suggest that it may not provide the necessary certainty to exclude the presence of microscopic residual disease altogether. Orel and coworkers [119] performed breast MR after excisional biopsy in 47 women with close or positive resection margins and correlated the MR findings with subsequent pathologic examination. In the postoperative setting, MR had a false-negative rate of 25%, and a negative predictive value of 61%. In comparison, preoperative MR is reported to have a false-negative rate of 5% to 20% and a negative predictive value of 77% to 95% [39,64,120–125]. Much of the subclinical residual disease in the breast is DCIS, and the negative predictive value of MR for DCIS is even lower than that reported for invasive carcinoma [32,37,38,64,123,126]. One reason for the higher false-negative rates of MR after surgery may be postoperative inflammation and edema. MR to select patients not requiring radiotherapy could be performed before surgery. However, a major constraint on the use of MR to exclude microscopic residual disease remains its spatial resolution. In studies of contrast-enhanced breast MR, the slice thickness is typically 2 mm (range 1 to 5 mm) with a gap of 0 to 2 mm between slices, so that 2 to 3 mm is the lowest theoretical threshold for MR sensitivity for disease detection. However, in clinical studies using MR imaging, the disease found is typically in the range of 4 to 8 mm in size [37,39,64,119–125]. The low specificity of breast MR makes further characterization of these very small lesions mandatory. The requirement for follow-up imaging could introduce an unacceptable delay between surgery and radiation, and pathologic confirmation would be difficult for very small lesions even with MR-guided needle biopsy. The threshold amount of microscopic disease in the breast, particularly DCIS, which is clinically significant, is uncertain. There is no doubt that

Table 6: **Local recurrence in prospective randomized trials in stage I-II breast cancer comparing breast-conserving surgery alone with breast-conserving surgery and radiation**

Trial	N	Tumor size (cm)	Tamoxifen (%)	Chemotherapy (%)	Local recurrence (%)		
					BCS	BCS+XRT	Follow-up (yr)
NSABP B-06 [2]	1,262	≤4 cm	0	37	39	14	20
Milan [101]	567	≤2.5	12	17	35	7	10
Uppsala-Örebro [102]	381	≤2	0	0	24	8.5	10
Ontario [103]	837	≤4	0	0	35	11	8
NSABP B-21 [104]	673	≤1	All	0	16.5	2.8[b]	8
Scottish [105]	585	≤4	73	26	24.5	5.8	6
GBSG [106]	173	≤2	0	0	29[a]	4[a]	5.9
	174	≤2	All		3[a]	3[a]	
British [107]	418	≤5	ER positive	ER negative	35	13	5
CALGB [108]	636	≤2	All	0	4	1	5
Canadian [109]	769	≤5	All	0	7.7	0.6	5
	611	≤2	All	0	5.9	0.4	5

Abbreviations: BCS, breast-conserving surgery; BCS+XRT, breast-conserving surgery and radiation; GBSG, German Breast Cancer Study Group; NSABP, National Surgical Adjuvant Breast and Bowel Project; CALGB, Cancer and Leukemia Group B.
[a] Crude results.
[b] 9.3% in patients not treated with tamoxifen.

the use of MR would allow the identification of some, but not all, tumor foci not visualized with mammography and ultrasonography. However, whether its use would allow a significant reduction in the number of patients requiring radiotherapy is uncertain given the substantial false-positive rates seen with MR.

The number of patients who may potentially benefit from MR is reduced further by improvements in the ability to identify patients at low risk for local recurrence without radiation using clinicopathologic selection factors. Factors that are associated with a higher risk of local recurrence in the absence of radiation include an extensive intraductal component, T2 tumor size, age less than 55 years, positive nodes, lymphovascular invasion, and invasive lobular histology [101–103,105,107]. These exclusion criteria can be identified without the use of breast MR. In a randomized trial of postoperative tamoxifen with or without radiation [108], eligible patients were those age 70 years or greater, with T1 tumors that were estrogen receptor (ER) positive, clinically negative nodes, and negative margins. The 5-year local recurrence rates were 4% with tamoxifen and 1% with tamoxifen and radiation. In a similar trial with more liberal entry criteria, T1/T2 node negative breast cancer patients older than 50 years were selected randomly to receive tamoxifen alone or tamoxifen and radiation [109]. The 5-year rates of local recurrence were approximately 1% with radiation and 8% without radiation. These studies found that although the use of clinicopathologic criteria has not been sufficient to identify a patient subgroup without *any* benefit from radiation, some subsets of patients with very low risks for local recurrence in the first 5 years after diagnosis can currently be identified.

Partial breast irradiation

The use of radiation therapy limited to the region of the tumor bed, or partial breast irradiation (PBI) is currently a subject of great interest. PBI is intended to improve the use and convenience of radiation therapy as a part of breast conservation by reducing the 6- to 6½ -week treatment time required for standard radiation to 5 days or less, while maintaining all, or most, of the proven efficacy of whole-breast irradiation. One requirement for PBI to be successful is that radiation therapy must not be necessary to the quadrants of the breast that are not involved by the primary tumor. However, unlike omission of radiation altogether, PBI has the potential to treat microscopic residual disease in close proximity to the tumor bed—disease known to be present commonly from pathologic studies [56,62,63,112–118, 127]. Techniques of PBI include interstitial multicatheter brachytherapy, Mammosite balloon catheter brachytherapy, or external beam radiation. These techniques treat approximately 1.5 to 2 cm of tissue around the lumpectomy cavity to the planned definitive dose of radiation. The occurrence of two thirds to three quarters of local recurrences after BCT in the original tumor quadrant supports the conceptual basis of PBI [24,26,75, 76]. Other reasons for increased interest in PBI include ease of use and clinical trial data showing very good early results in carefully selected patients.

Clinical experience with PBI has resulted in few local recurrences, although the length of follow-up in most studies is fairly short (Table 7) [128–136]. These favorable outcomes have been achieved using clinicopathologic selection factors to identify small, unifocal cancers without an extensive intraductal component. The potential of MR before treatment to improve on these selection criteria is uncertain. Wazer and coworkers [136] reported a study of PBI in patients with T1/T2 invasive ductal cancer, margins ≥1 mm, and 0 to 3 nodes positive without extracapsular extension. In 32 women followed up a median of 33 months, a single local recurrence outside of the implanted area was observed. Arthur and colleagues[128] reported the results of PBI in 44 patients with unifocal disease ≤4 cm, EIC negative, negative resection margins, and 0 to 3 nodes positive without extracapsular extension. After a median follow-up of 42 months, there were no local recurrences. In the study of Vicini and coauthors [135] 199 patients were treated with PBI. Selection criteria

Table 7: **Local recurrence in trials of partial breast brachytherapy**

Study	No. of patients	Median follow-up (mo)	Local recurrence (%)
Vicini et al [134]	793	7	<1
Polgar et al [133]	46	30	0
Wazer et al [136]	32	33	3
Arthur et al [128]	44	42	0
Kuske et al [130]	99	44	3
Vicini et al [135]	199	65	1
King et al [129]	50	75	2
Polgár et al [132]	45	81	9
Perera et al [131]	39	91	16

were age less than 40 years, tumor size ≤ 3 cm, non-lobular histology, margins greater than 2 mm, no EIC, and negative nodes. The 5-year cumulative incidence of local failure was 1% after a median follow-up of 65 months. Kuske and coauthors [130] reported the initial outcomes of a Radiation Therapy Oncology Group (RTOG) phase II trial of brachytherapy for patients with nonlobular tumors ≤ 3 cm, without an EIC, with 0 to 3 positive nodes, and negative margins. The 4-year actuarial rate of breast and nodal recurrences were both 3%. Polgár and coworkers [132] reported a phase I/II study of PBI for T1 tumors without lobular histology or an extensive in situ component. The 7-year local recurrence rate was 9%. In their subsequent phase III study assigning patients randomly to brachytherapy alone versus whole breast irradiation, the 3-year cause-specific and relapse-free survival rates were equal [133]. These findings suggest that appropriate candidates for PBI can be selected using conventional imaging and clinicopathologic selection factors. Based on the available data, MR is unlikely to have a clinically significant impact in reducing early local recurrence rates or to be cost effective unless larger studies document recurrence rates substantially higher than those observed in these initial studies.

The NSABP and the RTOG are now conducting a phase III randomized study, testing PBI against whole-breast radiation therapy, with endpoints of local control, survival, and quality of life. MR is a not part of the eligibility requirements or follow-up schedule for this study. However, entry criteria are fairly liberal and include patients with age ≥ 18 years, stage 0 to II breast cancer, tumor size ≤ 3 cm, 0 to 3 positive nodes, and a negative surgical margin. This study will provide definitive information on whether clinicopathologic selection criteria are able to define a large patient subset suitable for partial breast irradiation.

Summary

Experience with BCT has found that although subclinical multifocality/centricity is common in women who have localized breast cancer, extremely high rates of local control can be achieved in patients treated with radiotherapy and adjuvant systemic therapy. MR is a sensitive imaging modality that allows the detection of some of this subclinical disease. Unfortunately, the use of MR has the potential to result in unnecessary mastectomies, because contraindications to BCT owing to multicentricity or extensive multifocality are based on studies in which this disease was of sufficient volume to be detected by clinical examination or mammography. The selection of patients for BCT is a problem that has been solved for 95% of breast cancer patients. The addition of MR to this process will result in added costs and a prolongation of the time from initial diagnosis to definitive treatment. The lack of specificity of MR has the potential to result in many biopsies before definitive therapy, a factor known to cause women to opt for mastectomy [39]. In the absence of a clinical need, there seems to be little rationale for using MR in this way. An area of far greater clinical interest is the development of methods to select patients, particularly younger women, who do not require whole-breast irradiation. Here there is a strong rationale for the use of MR. Whether MR has sufficient resolution to identify patients who do not require any radiation is an open question as is the utility of MR in selecting patients for partial breast irradiation. There has already been widespread diffusion of MR into clinical use in spite of a lack of evidence to support improvement in patient outcomes. These questions will only be answered through prospective, randomized trials performed by collaborative groups of clinicians and radiologists.

References

[1] Arriagada R, Le MG, Rochard F, et al. Conservative treatment versus mastectomy in early breast cancer: patterns of failure with 15 years of follow-up data. Institut Gustave-Roussy Breast Cancer Group. J Clin Oncol 1996;14:1558.

[2] Fisher B, Anderson S, Bryant J, et al. Twenty-year follow-up of a randomized trial comparing total mastectomy, lumpectomy, and lumpectomy plus irradiation for the treatment of invasive breast cancer. N Engl J Med 2002;347: 1233.

[3] Veronesi U, Cascinelli N, Mariani L, et al. Twenty-year follow-up of a randomized study comparing breast-conserving surgery with radical mastectomy for early breast cancer. N Engl J Med 2002;347:1227.

[4] van Dongen J, Voogd AC, Fentiman IS, et al. Long-term results of a randomized trial comparing breast-conserving therapy with mastectomy: European Organization for Research and Treatment of Cancer 10801 trial. J Natl Cancer Inst 2000;92:1143.

[5] Poggi MM, Danforth DN, Sciuto LC, et al. Eighteen-year results in the treatment of early breast carcinoma with mastectomy versus breast conservation therapy: the National Cancer Institute Randomized Trial. Cancer 2003;98:697.

[6] Blichert-Toft M, Rose C, Andersen JA, et al. Danish randomized trial comparing breast conservation therapy with mastectomy: six years of life-table analysis. Danish Breast Cancer Cooperative Group. J Natl Cancer Inst Monogr 1992; 11:19–25.

[7] Morrow M, Schmidt R, Hassett C. Patient selection for breast conservation therapy with magnification mammography. Surgery 1995;118: 621.

[8] Winchester DP, Cox JD. Standards for breast-conservation treatment. CA Cancer J Clin 1992; 42:134.

[9] Morrow M, Strom EA, Bassett LW, et al. Standard for breast conservation therapy in the management of invasive breast carcinoma. CA Cancer J Clin 2002;52:277.

[10] Morrow M, Strom EA, Bassett LW, et al. Standard for the management of ductal carcinoma in situ of the breast (DCIS). CA Cancer J Clin 2002;52:256.

[11] Morrow M, Bucci C, Rademaker A. Medical contraindications are not a major factor in the underutilization of breast conserving therapy. J Am Coll Surg 1998;186:269.

[12] Morrow M, Schmidt RA, Bucci C. Breast conservation for mammographically occult carcinoma. Ann Surg 1998;227:502.

[13] Kearney TJ, Morrow M. Effect of reexcision on the success of breast-conserving surgery. Ann Surg Oncol 1995;2:303.

[14] Yeatman TJ, Cantor AB, Smith TJ, et al. Tumor biology of infiltrating lobular carcinoma. Implications for management. Ann Surg 1995;222: 549.

[15] Hussien M, Lioe TF, Finnegan J, et al. Surgical treatment for invasive lobular carcinoma of the breast. Breast 2003;12:23.

[16] Arpino G, Bardou VJ, Clark GM, et al. Infiltrating lobular carcinoma of the breast: tumor characteristics and clinical outcome. Breast Cancer Res 2004;6:R149.

[17] Morrow M, Keeney K, Scholtens D, et al. Selecting patients for breast conserving therapy: the importance of lobular histology. Cancer 2006; 106(12):2563–8.

[18] Freedman G, Fowble B, Hanlon A, et al. Patients with early stage invasive cancer with close or positive margins treated with conservative surgery and radiation have an increased risk of breast recurrence that is delayed by adjuvant systemic therapy. Int J Radiat Oncol Biol Phys 1999;44:1005.

[19] Park CC, Mitsumori M, Nixon A, et al. Outcome at 8 years after breast-conserving surgery and radiation therapy for invasive breast cancer: influence of margin status and systemic therapy on local recurrence. J Clin Oncol 2000;18:1668.

[20] Smitt MC, Nowels KW, Zdeblick MJ, et al. The importance of the lumpectomy surgical margin status in long-term results of breast conservation. Cancer 1995;76:259.

[21] Peterson ME, Schultz DJ, Reynolds C, et al. Outcomes in breast cancer patients relative to margin status after treatment with breast-conserving surgery and radiation therapy: the University of Pennsylvania experience. Int J Radiat Oncol Biol Phys 1999;43:1029.

[22] Wazer DE, Schmidt-Ullrich RK, Ruthazer R, et al. Factors determining outcome for breast-conserving irradiation with margin-directed dose escalation to the tumor bed. Int J Radiat Oncol Biol Phys 1998;40:851.

[23] Wapnir I, Anderson S, Mamounas E, et al. Survival after IBTR in NSABP Node Negative Protocols B-13, B-14, B-19, B-20 and B-23 [abstract 517]. J Clin Oncol 2005;23:8s.

[24] Freedman GM, Hanlon AL, Fowble BL, et al. Recursive partitioning identifies patients at high and low risk for ipsilateral tumor recurrence after breast-conserving surgery and radiation. J Clin Oncol 2002;20:4015.

[25] Kini VR, Vicini FA, Frazier R, et al. Mammographic, pathologic, and treatment-related factors associated with local recurrence in patients with early-stage breast cancer treated with breast conserving therapy. Int J Radiat Oncol Biol Phys 1999;43:341.

[26] Santiago RJ, Wu L, Harris E, et al. Fifteen-year results of breast-conserving surgery and definitive irradiation for stage I and II breast carcinoma: The University of Pennsylvania experience. Int J Rad Oncol Biol Phys 2004;58:233.

[27] Pass H, Vicini FA, Kestin LL, et al. Changes in management techniques and patterns of disease recurrence over time in patients with breast carcinoma treated with breast-conserving therapy at a single institution. Cancer 2004;101:713.

[28] Ernst MF, Voogd AC, Coebergh JW, et al. Using loco-regional recurrence as an indicator of the quality of breast cancer treatment. Eur J Cancer 2004;40:487.

[29] Fisher B, Anderson S, Fisher ER, et al. Significance of ipsilateral breast tumour recurrence after lumpectomy. Lancet 1991;338:327.

[30] Baum M, Budzar AU, Cuzick J, et al. Anastrozole alone or in combination with tamoxifen versus tamoxifen alone for adjuvant treatment of postmenopausal women with early breast cancer: first results of the ATAC randomised trial. Lancet 2002;359:2131.

[31] Orel SG, Schnall MD, Powell CM, et al. Staging of suspected breast cancer: effect of MR imaging and MR-guided biopsy. Radiology 1995;196: 115.

[32] Boetes C, Mus RD, Holland R, et al. Breast tumors: comparative accuracy of MR imaging relative to mammography and US for demonstrating extent. Radiology 1995;197:743.

[33] Mumtaz H, Hall-Craggs MA, Davidson T, et al. Staging of symptomatic primary breast cancer with MR imaging. AJR Am J Roentgenol 1997; 169:417.

[34] Fischer U, Kopka L, Grabbe E. Breast carcinoma: effect of preoperative contrast-enhanced MR imaging on the therapeutic approach. Radiology 1999;213:881.

[35] Drew PJ, Chatterjee S, Turnbull LW, et al. Dynamic contrast enhanced magnetic resonance imaging of the breast is superior to triple

assessment for the pre-operative detection of multifocal breast cancer. Ann Surg Oncol 1999;6:599.

[36] Bedrosian I, Mick R, Orel SG, et al. Changes in the surgical management of patients with breast carcinoma based on preoperative magnetic resonance imaging. Cancer 2003;98: 468.

[37] Liberman L, Morris EA, Dershaw DD, et al. MR imaging of the ipsilateral breast in women with percutaneously proven breast cancer. AJR Am J Roentgenol 2003;180:901.

[38] Bluemke DA, Gatsonis CA, Chen MH, et al. Magnetic resonance imaging of the breast prior to biopsy. JAMA 2004;292:2735.

[39] Berg WA, Gutierrez L, NessAiver MS, et al. Diagnostic accuracy of mammography, clinical examination, US, and MR imaging in preoperative assessment of breast cancer. Radiology 2004; 233:830.

[40] Deurloo EE, Peterse JL, Rutgers EJ, et al. Additional breast lesions in patients eligible for breast-conserving therapy by MRI: impact on preoperative management and potential benefit of computerised analysis. Eur J Cancer 2005;41: 1393–401.

[41] Deurloo EE, Klein Zeggelink WF, Teertstra HJ, et al. Contrast-enhanced MRI in breast cancer patients eligible for breast-conserving therapy: complementary value for subgroups of patients. Eur Radiol 2006;16(3):692.

[42] Weinstein SP, Orel SG, Heller R, et al. MR imaging of the breast in patients with invasive lobular carcinoma. AJR Am J Roentgenol 2001;176: 399.

[43] Kneeshaw PJ, Turnbull LW, Smith A, et al. Dynamic contrast enhanced magnetic resonance imaging aids the surgical management of invasive lobular breast cancer. Eur J Surg Oncol 2003;29:32.

[44] Schelfout K, Van Goethem M, Kersschot E, et al. Preoperative breast MRI in patients with invasive lobular breast cancer. Eur Radiol 2004;14: 1209.

[45] Quan ML, Sclafani L, Heerdt AS, et al. Magnetic resonance imaging detects unsuspected disease in patients with invasive lobular cancer. Ann Surg Oncol 2003;10:1048.

[46] Munot K, Dall B, Achuthan R, et al. Role of magnetic resonance imaging in the diagnosis and single-stage surgical resection of invasive lobular carcinoma of the breast. Br J Surg 2002;89:1296.

[47] Winchester DJ, Chang HR, Graves TA, et al. A comparative analysis of lobular and ductal carcinoma of the breast: presentation, treatment, and outcomes. J Am Coll Surg 1998;186:416.

[48] Peiro G, Bornstein BA, Connolly JL, et al. The influence of infiltrating lobular carcinoma on the outcome of patients treated with breast-conserving surgery and radiation therapy. Breast Cancer Res Treat 2000;59:49.

[49] Santiago RJ, Harris EE, Qin L, et al. Similar long-term results of breast-conservation treatment for Stage I and II invasive lobular carcinoma compared with invasive ductal carcinoma of the breast. Cancer 2005;103:2447.

[50] Weiss MC, Fowble BL, Solin LJ, et al. Outcome of conservative therapy for invasive breast cancer by histologic subtype. Int J Radiat Oncol Biol Phys 1992;23:941.

[51] White JR, Gustafson GS, Wimbish K, et al. Conservative surgery and radiation therapy for infiltrating lobular carcinoma of the breast. The role of preoperative mammograms in guiding treatment. Cancer 1994;74:640.

[52] Molland JG, Donnellan M, Janu NC, et al. Infiltrating lobular carcinoma—a comparison of diagnosis, management and outcome with infiltrating duct carcinoma. Breast 2004;13:389.

[53] Tillman GF, Orel SG, Schnall MD, et al. Effect of breast magnetic resonance imaging on the clinical management of women with early-stage breast carcinoma. J Clin Oncol 2002;20:3413.

[54] Koida T, Kimura M, Yanagita Y, et al. Clinicopathological study of unilateral multiple breast cancer. Breast Cancer 2001;8:202.

[55] Qualheim RE, Gall EA. Breast carcinoma with multiple sites of origin. Cancer 1957;10:460.

[56] Rosen PP, Fracchia AA, Urban JA, et al. "Residual" mammary carcinoma following simulated partial mastectomy. Cancer 1975;35:739.

[57] Lagios MD. Multicentricity of breast carcinoma demonstrated by routine correlated serial subgross and radiographic examination. Cancer 1977;40:1726.

[58] Egan RL. Multicentric breast carcinomas: clinical-radiographic-pathologic whole organ studies and 10-year survival. Cancer 1982;49:1123.

[59] Schwartz GF, Patchesfsky AS, Feig SA, et al. Multicentricity of non-palpable breast cancer. Cancer 1980;45:2913.

[60] Vaidya JS, Vyas JJ, Chinoy RF, et al. Multicentricity of breast cancer: whole-organ analysis and clinical implications. Br J Cancer 1996; 74:820.

[61] Anastassiades O, Iakovou E, Stavridou N, et al. Multicentricity in breast cancer. A study of 366 cases. Am J Clin Pathol 1993;99:238.

[62] Holland R, Veling SH, Mravunac M, et al. Histologic multifocality of Tis, T1–2 breast carcinomas. Implications for clinical trials of breast-conserving surgery. Cancer 1985;56:979.

[63] Holland R, Connolly JL, Gelman R, et al. The presence of an extensive intraductal component following a limited excision correlates with prominent residual disease in the remainder of the breast. J Clin Oncol 1990;8:113.

[64] Sardanelli F, Giuseppetti GM, Panizza P, et al. Sensitivity of MRI versus mammography for detecting foci of multifocal multicentric breast cancer infatty and dense breasts using the whole-breast pathologic examination as a gold standard. Am J Roentgenol 2004;183:1149.

[65] Fischer U, Zachariae O, Baum F, et al. The influence of preoperative MRI of the breasts on recurrence rate in patients with breast cancer. Eur Radiol 2004;14:1725.

[66] Fisher B, Dignam J, Bryant J, et al. Five versus more than five years of tamoxifen therapy for breast cancer patients with negative lymph nodes and estrogen receptor-positive tumors. J Natl Cancer Inst 1996;88:1529.

[67] Dalberg K, Johansson H, Johansson U, et al. A randomized trial of long term adjuvant tamoxifen plus postoperative radiation therapy versus radiation therapy alone for patients with early stage breast carcinoma treated with breast-conserving surgery. Stockholm Breast Cancer Study Group. Cancer 1998;82:2204.

[68] Fisher B, Dignam J, Mamounas EP, et al. Sequential methotrexate and fluorouracil for the treatment of node-negative breast cancer patients with estrogen receptor-negative tumors: eight-year results from National Surgical Adjuvant Breast and Bowel Project (NSABP) B-13 and first report of findings from NSABP B-19 comparing methotrexate and fluorouracil with conventional cyclophosphamide, methotrexate, and fluorouracil. J Clin Oncol 1996;14:1982.

[69] Esserman L, Hylton N, Yassa L, et al. Utility of magnetic resonance imaging in the management of breast cancer: evidence for improved preoperative staging. J Clin Oncol 1999;17:110.

[70] Wallace AM, Daniel BL, Jeffrey SS, et al. Rates of reexcision for breast cancer after magnetic resonance imaging-guided bracket wire localization. J Am Coll Surg 2005;200:527.

[71] Staradub VL, Rademaker AW, Morrow M. Factors influencing outcomes for breast conservation therapy of mammographically detected malignancies. J Am Coll Surg 2003;196:518.

[72] Arriagada R, Le MG, Contesso G, et al. Predictive factors for local recurrence in 2006 patients with surgically resected small breast cancer. Ann Oncol 2002;13:1404.

[73] Bartelink H, Horiot JC, Poortmans P, et al. Recurrence rates after treatment of breast cancer with standard radiotherapy with or without additional radiation. N Engl J Med 2001;345:1378.

[74] Kroman N, Holtveg H, Wohlfahrt J, et al. Effect of breast-conserving therapy versus radical mastectomy on prognosis for young women with breast carcinoma. Cancer 2004;100:688.

[75] Galper S, Blood E, Gelman R, et al. Prognosis after local recurrence after conservative surgery and radiation for early-stage breast cancer. Int J Radiat Oncol Biol Phys 2005;61:348.

[76] Krauss DJ, Kestin LL, Mitchell C, et al. Changes in temporal patterns of local failure after breast-conserving therapy and their prognostic implications. Int J Radiat Oncol Biol Phys 2004;60:731.

[77] Smith TE, Lee D, Turner BC, et al. True recurrence vs. new primary ipsilateral breast tumor relapse: an analysis of clinical and pathologic differences and their implications in natural history, prognosis, and therapeutic management. Int J Radiat Oncol Biol Phys 2000;48:1281.

[78] Katz S, Lantz P, Janz N, et al. Patient involvement in surgery treatment decisions for breast cancer. J Clin Oncol 2005;23:5526–33.

[79] Chauvet B, Reynaud-Bougnoux A, Calais G, et al. Prognostic significance of breast relapse after conservative treatment in node-negative early breast cancer. Int J Radiat Oncol Biol Phys 1990;19:1125.

[80] Dalberg K, Mattsson A, Sandelin K, et al. Outcome of treatment for ipsilateral breast tumor recurrence in early-stage breast cancer. Breast Cancer Res Treat 1998;49:69.

[81] Francis M, Cakir B, Ung O, et al. Prognosis after breast recurrence following conservative surgery and radiotherapy in patients with node-negative breast cancer. Br J Surg 1999;86:1556.

[82] Haffty B, Fischer D, Beinfield M, et al. Prognosis following local recurrence in the conservatively treated breast cancer patient. Int J Radiat Oncol Biol Phys 1991;21:293.

[83] Stotter AT, McNeese MD, Ames FC, et al. Predicting the rate and extent of locoregional failure after breast conservation therapy for early breast cancer. Cancer 1989;64:2217.

[84] Voogd AC, van Tienhoven G, Peterse HL, et al. Local recurrence after breast conservation therapy for early stage breast carcinoma. Detection, treatment, and outcome in 266 patients. Cancer 1999;85:437.

[85] Fisher ER, Anderson S, Redmond C, et al. Ipsilateral breast tumor recurrence and survival following lumpectomy and irradiation: pathologic findings from NSABP protocol B-06. Semin Surg Oncol 1992;8:161.

[86] Gage I, Schnitt SJ, Recht A, et al. Skin recurrences after breast-conserving therapy for early-stage breast cancer. J Clin Oncol 1998;16:480.

[87] Philpotts LE, Lee CH, Haffty BG, et al. Mammographic findings of recurrent breast cancer after lumpectomy and radiation therapy: comparison with the primary tumor. Radiology 1996;201:767.

[88] Touboul E, Buffat L, Belkacémi Y, et al. Local recurrences and distant metastases after breast-conserving surgery and radiation therapy for early breast cancer. Int J Radiat Oncol Biol Phys 1999;43:25.

[89] Veronesi U, Marubini E, Del Vecchio M, et al. Local recurrences and distant metastases after conservative breast cancer treatments: partly independent events. J Natl Cancer Inst 1995;87:19.

[90] Jacobson JA, Danforth DN, Cowan KH, et al. Ten-year results of a comparison of conservation with mastectomy in the treatment of stage I and II breast cancer. N Engl J Med 1995;332:907.

[91] Kurtz JM, Spitalier J-M, Amalric R, et al. The prognostic significance of late local recurrence after breast-conserving therapy. Int J Radiat Oncol Biol Phys 1990;18:87.

[92] Salvadori B, Marubini E, Miceli R, et al. Reoperation for locally recurrent breast cancer in patients previously treated with conservative surgery. Br J Surg 1999;86:84.

[93] Fortin A, Larochelle M, Laverdière J, et al. Local failure is responsible for the decrease in survival for patients with breast cancer treated with conservative surgery and postoperative radiotherapy. J Clin Oncol 1999;17:101.

[94] van Tienhoven G, Voogd AC, Peterse JL, et al. Prognosis after treatment for loco-regional recurrence after mastectomy or breast conserving therapy in two randomised trials (EORTC 10801 and DBCG-82TM). Eur J Cancer 1999; 35:32.

[95] Deutsch M. Repeat high dose partial breast irradiation after lumpectomy for in-breast tumor recurrences following initial lumpectomy and radiotherapy. Int J Rad Oncol Biol Phys 1998; 42:255.

[96] Kurtz JM, Jacquemier J, Amalric R, et al. Is breast conservation after local recurrence feasible? Eur J Cancer 1991;27:240.

[97] Fourquet A, Campana F, Zafrani B, et al. Prognostic factors of breast recurrence in the conservative management of early breast cancer: a 25-year follow-up. Int J Radiat Oncol Biol Phys 1989;17:719.

[98] Galper S, Blood E, Gelman R, et al. Prognosis after local recurrence after conservative surgery and radiation for early-stage breast cancer. Int J Radiat Oncol Biol Phys 2005;61:348.

[99] Haffty BG, Reiss M, Beinfield M, et al. Ipsilateral breast tumor recurrence as a predictor of distant disease: implications for systemic therapy at the time of local relapse. J Clin Oncol 1996;14:52.

[100] Katz SJ, Lantz PM, Janz NK, et al. Patterns and correlates of local therapy for women with ductal carcinoma-in-situ. J Clin Oncol 2005;23: 3001.

[101] Veronesi U, Marubini E, Mariani L, et al. Radiotherapy after breast-conserving surgery in small breast carcinoma: long-term results of a randomized trial. Ann Oncol 2001;12:997.

[102] Liljegren G, Holmberg L, Bergh J, et al. 10 year results after sector resection with or without postoperative radiotherapy for stage I breast cancer: a randomized trial. J Clin Oncol 1999; 17:2326.

[103] Clark RM, Whelan T, Levine M, et al. Randomized clinical trial of breast irradiation following lumpectomy and axillary dissection for node-negative breast cancer: an update. J Natl Cancer Inst 1996;88:1659.

[104] Fisher B, Bryant J, Dignam JJ, et al. Tamoxifen, radiation therapy, or both for prevention of ipsilateral breast tumor recurrence after lumpectomy in women with invasive breast cancers of one centimeter or less. J Clin Oncol 2002; 20:4141–9.

[105] Forrest AP, Stewart HJ, Everington D, et al. Randomised controlled trial of conservation therapy for breast cancer: 6-year analysis of the Scottish trial. Lancet 1996;348:708.

[106] Winzer KJ, Sauer R, Sauerbrei W, et al. Radiation therapy after breast-conserving surgery: first results of a randomised clinical trial in patients with low risk of recurrence. Eur J Cancer 2004;40:998.

[107] Renton SC, Gazet J-C, Ford HT, et al. The importance of the resection margin in conservative surgery for breast cancer. Eur J Surg Oncol 1996;22:17.

[108] Hughes KS, Schnaper LA, Berry D, et al. Lumpectomy plus tamoxifen with or without irradiation in women 70 years of age or older with early breast cancer. N Engl J Med 2004;351:971.

[109] Fyles AW, McCready DR, Manchul LA, et al. Tamoxifen with or without breast irradiation in women 50 years of age or older with early breast cancer. N Engl J Med 2004;351:963.

[110] Lim M, Nixon AJ, Gelman R, et al. A prospective study of conservative surgery (CS) alone without radiotherapy (RT) in selected patients with stage I breast cancer [abstract]. Breast Cancer Res Treat 1999;57:34.

[111] Schnitt SJ, Hayman J, Gelman R, et al. A prospective study of conservative surgery alone in the treatment of selected patients with stage I breast cancer. Cancer 1996;77:1094.

[112] Beron PJ, Horwitz EM, Martinez AA, et al. Pathologic and mammographic findings predicting the adequacy of tumor excision before breast-conserving therapy. Am J Radiol 1996;167:1409.

[113] Gwin JL, Eisenberg BL, Hoffman JP, et al. Incidence of gross and microscopic carcinoma in specimens from patients with breast cancer after re-excision lumpectomy. Ann Surg 1993;218:729.

[114] Schnitt SJ, Connolly JL, Khettry U, et al. Pathologic findings on re-excision of the primary site in breast cancer patients considered for treatment by primary radiation therapy. Cancer 1987; 59:675.

[115] Solin LJ, Fowble B, Martz K, et al. Results of re-excisional biopsy of the primary tumor in preparation for definitive irradiation of patients with early stage breast cancer. Int J Radiat Oncol Biol Phys 1986;12:721.

[116] Wazer DE, Schmidt-Ullrich RK, Ruthazer R, et al. The influence of age and extensive intraductal component histology upon breast lumpectomy margin assessment as a predictor of residual tumor. Int J Radiat Oncol Biol Phys 1999;45:885.

[117] Faverly DRG, Hendriks JHCL, Holland R. Breast carcinomas of limited extent. Frequency, radiologic-pathologic characteristics, and surgical margin requirements. Cancer 2001;91:647.

[118] Holland R, Faverly DRG. Whole-organ studies. In: Silverstein M, editor. Ductal carcinoma in

situ of the breast. Baltimore: Williams & Wilkins; 1997. p. 233.

[119] Orel SG, Reynolds C, Schnall MD, et al. Breast carcinoma: MR imaging before re-excisional biopsy. Radiology 1997;205:429.

[120] Boetes C, Barentsz JO, Mus RD, et al. MR characterization of suspicious breast lesions with a gadolinium-enhanced turboFLASH subtraction technique. Radiology 1994;193:777.

[121] Gilles R, Guinebretière JM, Lucidarme O, et al. Nonpalpable breast tumors: diagnosis with contrast-enhanced subtraction dynamic MR imaging. Radiology 1994;191:625.

[122] Harms SE, Flamig DP, Hesley KL, et al. MR imaging of the breast with rotating delivery of excitation off resonance: clinical experience with pathologic correlation. Radiology 1993;187:493.

[123] Hata T, Takahashi H, Watanabe K, et al. Magnetic resonance imaging for preoperative evaluation of breast cancer: a comparative study with mammography and ultrasonography. J Am Coll Surg 2004;198:190.

[124] Olson JA Jr, Morris EA, Van Zee KJ, et al. Magnetic resonance imaging facilitates breast conservation for occult breast cancer. Ann Surg Oncol 2000;7:411.

[125] Stomper PC, Herman S, Klippenstein DL, et al. Suspect breast lesions: findings at dynamic gadolinium-enhanced MR imaging correlated with mammographic and pathologic features. Radiology 1995;197:387.

[126] Ikeda O, Nishimura R, Miyayama H, et al. Magnetic resonance evaluation of the presence of an extensive intraductal component in breast cancer. Acta Radiol 2004;45:721.

[127] Frazier TG, Wong RWY, Rose D. Implications of accurate pathologic margins in the treatment of primary breast cancer. Arch Surg 1989; 124:37.

[128] Arthur DW, Koo D, Zwicker RD, et al. Partial breast brachytherapy after lumpectomy: low-dose-rate and high-dose-rate experience. Int J Radiat Oncol Biol Phys 2003;56:681.

[129] King TA, Bolton JS, Kuske RR, et al. Long-term results of wide-field brachytherapy as the sole method of radiation therapy after segmental mastectomy for T(is, 1,2) breast cancer. Am J Surg 2000;180:299.

[130] Kuske RR, Winter K, Arthur DW, et al. A phase II trial of brachytherapy alone following lumpectomy for stage I or II breast cancer: Initial outcomes of RTOG 9517. J Clin Oncol 2004; 23:18.

[131] Perera F, Yu E, Engel J, et al. Patterns of breast recurrence in a pilot study of brachytherapy confined to the lumpectomy site for early breast cancer with six years' minimum follow-up. Int J Radiat Oncol Biol Phys 2003;57:1239.

[132] Polgár C, Major T, Fodor J, et al. High-dose-rate brachytherapy alone versus whole breast radiotherapy with or without tumor bed boost after breast-conserving surgery: seven-year results of a comparative study. Int J Rad Oncol Biol Phys 2004;60:1173.

[133] Polgár C, Sulyok Z, Fodor J, et al. Sole brachytherapy of the tumor bed after conservative surgery for T1 breast cancer: five-year results of a phase I–II study and initial findings of a randomized phase III trial. J Surg Oncol 2002; 80:121.

[134] Vicini FA, Beitsch P, Quiet C, et al. First analysis of patient demographics and technical reproducibility by the American Society of Breast Surgeons (ASBS) MammoSite breast brachytherapy registry trial in 801 patients treated with accelerated partial breast irradiation (APBI) [abstract 4070]. Br Cancer Res Treat 2004;88(1):1–253.

[135] Vicini FA, Kestin L, Chen P, et al. Limited-field radiation therapy in the management of early-stage breast cancer. J Natl Cancer Inst 2003; 95:1205.

[136] Wazer DE, Berle L, Graham R, et al. Preliminary results of a phase I/II study of HDR brachytherapy alone for T1/T2 breast cancer. Int J Rad Oncol Biol Phys 2002;53:889.

MAGNETIC
RESONANCE
IMAGING CLINICS

Magn Reson Imaging Clin N Am 14 (2006) 379–381

MR Imaging Evaluation of Cancer Extent: Is There Clinical Relevance?

Mitchell Schnall, MD, PhD

■ References

The assessment of the extent of cancer in an affected breast is an important factor in the selection of women for breast conservation. It is well known from the work of Holland and colleagues [1] that up to 63% of the patients with clinical and mammographic assessment of having unifocal breast cancer have additional malignant foci in the ipsilateral breast. Holland and colleagues [1] reported cancer greater than 2 cm from the index lesions in 43% of women presenting with breast cancer. This includes a 16% incidence of invasive cancer and a 27% incidence of ductal carcinoma in situ (DCIS) greater than 2 cm from the index lesion. The tendency for breast cancer to present as multifocal and multicentric disease results in unacceptable local failure rates for lumpectomy alone of up to 40% [2–5].

The use of adjuvant radiation therapy is the clinical standard for breast conservation therapy (BCT). Although it has a major role in reducing local recurrence, the reported rate of ipsilateral breast cancer in breast cancer recurrence varies and has been reported to be as high as 19% at 10 years in randomized studies [3,6,7]. In addition, multiple retrospective case series report local recurrence higher than 10% for BCT [8,9]. Among the major factors influencing the recurrence rate, the most significant seems to be the extent of cancer remaining in the breast after lumpectomy. This is manifested by higher recurrence rates in women with an extensive intraductal component, positive or close surgical margins, and mammographically

or clinically detected multicentric disease [10]. In developing standards for the selection of patients for breast conservation, a joint task force from the American College of Surgery, American College of Pathology, and American College of Radiology recommends that mammographically detected multicentric disease be considered a contraindication to BCT [10]. Further, positive surgical margins after a reasonable number of attempts at surgical excision is also considered a contraindication to BCT. Clearly, there is recognition that gross tumor remaining in the breast after surgical excision increases the risk of recurrence and should influence treatment decisions.

Multiple studies have shown that MR imaging detects additional foci of cancer in up to 30% of women presenting with mammographically detected unifocal breast cancer [11–16]. Perhaps the best data illustrating the ability of MR imaging to detect additional foci of cancer remote from the index lesion come from the multicenter trial conducted by the International Breast MR Imaging Consortium (IBMC 6883) [17]. This study used a clear standard that required disease to be greater than 2 cm separated from the index lesion to be classified as a distinct focus of disease. Although this is not the traditional definition of multicentricity that requires lesions to be in different quadrants, the "2-cm rule" is better suited to three-dimensional (3D) imaging techniques, where precise 3D localization is possible. The separate quadrant

Department of Radiology, Hospital of the University of Pennsylvania, 3400 Spruce Street, Philadelphia, PA 19104, USA
E-mail address: schnall@oasis.rad.upenn.edu

1064-9689/06/$ – see front matter © 2006 Elsevier Inc. All rights reserved.
mri.theclinics.com

doi:10.1016/j.mric.2006.07.005

definition was developed with the projection image technique of mammography in mind. Using the 2-cm rule, additional cancer foci were detected mammographically in 7.5% of 426 women and by MR imaging in 18% of 426 women who presented with primary breast cancer. This cohort was selected from those women with a cancer diagnosis entering a diagnostic study, and therefore represents a general cancer population not biased toward advanced cancer. The recommendations would suggest that the women with mammographically detected additional cancer foci not be offered BCT. The 7% rate of mammogram detection in the IBMC 6883 study is consistent with reported rates of mammographically detected multicentricity.

The significance of the detection of an additional 10% of women with additional cancer foci by MR imaging needs to be considered. Studies of the impact of MR imaging on local recurrence are difficult. There is only a single published study aimed at retrospectively comparing recurrence rates in a cohort of women treated with BCT after being staged with MR imaging with those in a cohort of women who had not been staged with MR imaging [18]. Unfortunately the non-MR imaging–staged cohort seems to be biased toward more aggressive lesions based on higher rates of positive nodes and metastatic disease at presentation. Therefore, the decreased recurrence rate of the MR imaging–staged group may be partially related to the differences in tumor biology. Further, prospective randomized studies have been difficult to develop because of concern over compliance with randomization and accrual. Even if initiated today, results are not going to be available for many years. Thus, in the absence of strong clinical data, we are left with projecting the significance of MR imaging only based on the characteristics of the additional cancer foci detected.

It is suggested that the MR imaging–detected cancer is subclinical because of the fact that the cancer has not grown enough to become detectable by mammography. If we compare the additional cancer foci detected by mammography with those detected by MR imaging exclusively, however, they appear strikingly similar. Table 1 illustrates the characteristics of the mammographically and MR imaging only–detected additional cancer foci.

Both modalities detect similar rates of invasive cancer, and both detect lesions with a median size of approximately 1.0 cm. In addition, the grades of the additional cancer foci detected by the two techniques are similar. Thus, it is hard to understand how the mammogram detecting additional cancer foci can have different significance than the MR imaging–detected cancer.

It is generally held that radiotherapy cannot control foci of cancer greater than 1 cm. If the median size of the additional cancer foci detected by MR imaging alone is 1.1 cm, approximately 5% of women would have occult cancer detected by MR imaging that would not be controlled by radiotherapy. Thus, applying MR imaging as part of the preoperative evaluation of the ipsilateral breast in women presenting with breast cancer considering BCT has the potential to reduce the local recurrence rate by at least 5%. Applying conventional treatment paradigms, this would be achieved with an increase in the mastectomy rate by 5% to 10% depending on whether a size criterion is applied to developing treatment recommendations for women with MR imaging only–detected additional cancer foci.

Another concern frequently raised is the number of MR imaging false-positive findings leading to many unnecessary biopsies. Again, review of the IBMC 6883 data suggest that in the setting of determining the extent of primary breast cancer, the false-positive rate is relatively low at 28% in trained hands, which is likely partially attributable to the high pretest probability of disease. This false-positive rate is acceptable when consideration is given to another value that MR imaging provides in the preoperative setting. By better demonstrating the size of the primary lesion and detecting an extensive intraductal component, MR imaging can reduce the reliance on evaluation of the lumpectomy specimen to stage a patient accurately, and thus reduce the number of operative procedures for some women.

A final consideration relates to the changing technology used for BCT. The development of more targeted approaches of radiotherapy using intensity-modulated radiation therapy (IMRT) and brachytherapy reduces morbidity but does not provide the dose distribution used in the early studies of BCT. Thus, applying these techniques places

Table 1: **Characteristics of additional cancer foci**

	Mammographically detected IL (+/− MR imaging) (n = 17)	MR imaging only detected IL (n = 41)
Invasive (%)	76.5%	78%
Size (median)	12 mm	11 mm
Grade 2 or 3 (%) (invasive)	70%	84%
Grade 3 (%) (invasive)	0%	35%

greater emphasis on the need to identify additional cancer foci. Finally, we need to look toward the future of BCT. There are a number of ablation technologies that are under development for the treatment of breast cancer. Many paradigms can be envisioned, including ablation of all MR imaging–detected disease to expand the population of women eligible for BCT.

In conclusion, the traditional methods for selecting women for BCT, coupled with adjuvant radiation therapy, have reduced recurrence rates of BCT to acceptable levels. These recurrence rates are still significant, however. They may be further affected by the application of more anatomically targeted radiation therapy. The MR imaging only additional cancer foci seem to be significant based on size and histology. The false-positive rates for MR imaging performed by experienced radiologists seem to be modest. Preoperative MR imaging should theoretically reduce the local failure rate of BCT by at least 5%, with only a modest increase in the mastectomy rate. The evolution of BCT to include more targeted radiation therapy and ablation should place an even larger emphasis on accurate tumor localization and has the potential to allow BCT to become more prevalent and effective.

References

[1] Holland R, Veling SHJ, Mravunac M, et al. Histologic multifocality of Tis, T1-2 breast carcinomas: implications for clinical trials of breast-conserving surgery. Cancer 1985;56:979–90.

[2] Veronesi U, Luini A, Galimberti V, et al. Conservation approaches for the management of Stage I/II carcinoma of the breast: Milan Cancer Institute trials. World J Surg 1994;18:70–5.

[3] Fisher B, Anderson S, Redmond CK, et al. Reanalysis and results after 12 years of follow-up in a randomized clinical trial comparing total mastectomy with lumpectomy with or without irradiation in the treatment of breast cancer. N Engl J Med 1995;333:1456–61.

[4] Veronesi U, Luini A, Del Vecchio M, et al. Radiotherapy after breast preserving surgery in women with localized cancer of the breast. N Engl J Med 1993;328:1587–91.

[5] Spooner D, Morrison JM, Oates GD, et al. The role of radiotherapy in early breast cancer (Stage I). A West Midlands Breast Group prospective randomized collaborative study (BR 3002). Breast 1995;4:231–4.

[6] Jacobson JA, Danforth DN, Cowan KH, et al. Ten-year results of a comparison of conservation with mastectomy in the treatment of Stage I and II breast cancer. N Engl J Med 1995;332:907–11.

[7] van Dongen JA, Voogd AC, Fentiman IS, et al. Long-term results of a randomized trial comparing breast-conserving therapy with mastectomy: European Organization for Research and Treatment of Cancer 10801 Trial. J Natl Cancer Inst 2000;92:1143–50.

[8] Fowble B, Solin LJ, Schultz DJ, et al. Ten-year results of conservative surgery and radiation for Stage I and II breast cancer. Int J Radiat Oncol Biol Phys 1991;21:269–77.

[9] Haffty BG, Goldberg NB, Rose M, et al. Conservative surgery with radiation therapy in clinical Stage I and II breast cancer: results of a 20-year experience. Arch Surg 1989;124:1266–70.

[10] Morrow M, Strom EA, Bassett LW, et al. American College of Radiology; American College of Surgeons; Society of Surgical Oncology; College of American Pathology. Standard for breast conservation therapy in the management of invasive breast carcinoma. CA Cancer J Clin 2002;52:277–300.

[11] Harms SE, Flamig DP, Hesley KL, et al. MR imaging of the breast with rotating delivery of excitation off resonance: clinical experience with pathologic correlation. Radiology 1993;187:493–501.

[12] Orel S, Schnall M, Powell C, et al. Staging of suspected breast cancer: effect of MR imaging and MR guided biopsy. Radiology 1995;196:115–22.

[13] Fischer U, Kopka L, Grabbe E. Breast carcinoma: effect of preoperative contrast enhanced MR imaging on the therapeutic approach. Radiology 1999;213:881–8.

[14] Boetes C, Mus RD, Holland R, et al. Breast tumors: comparative accuracy of MR imaging relative to mammography and US for demonstrating extent. Radiology 1995;197:743–7.

[15] Mumtaz H, Hall-Craggs MA, Davidson T, et al. Staging of symptomatic primary breast cancer with MR imaging. AJR Am J Roentgenol 1997;169:417–24.

[16] Kramer S, Schulz-Wendtland R, Hagedorn K, et al. Magnetic resonance imaging and its role in the diagnosis of multicentric breast cancer. Anticancer Res 1998;18:2163–4.

[17] Schnall MD, Blume J, Bluemke DA, et al. MRI detection of distinct incidental cancer in women with primary breast cancer studied in IBMC 6883. J Surg Oncol 2005;92(1):32–8.

[18] Fischer U, Zachariae O, Baum F, et al. The influence of preoperative MRI of the breasts on recurrence rate in patients with breast cancer. Eur Radiol 2004;14(10):1725–31.

MAGNETIC
RESONANCE
IMAGING CLINICS

Magn Reson Imaging Clin N Am 14 (2006) 383–389

MR Imaging for Assessment of Breast Cancer Response to Neoadjuvant Chemotherapy

Nola Hylton, PhD

- ■ MR imaging for assessing residual disease
- ■ MR imaging for monitoring tumor response
- ■ References

The NSABP B-18 trial, a randomized study comparing pre- and postoperative chemotherapy in women with operable breast cancer, found no statistically significant difference in overall or disease-free survival between these two groups [1,2]. Several smaller randomized trials have had similar results [3,4] or have found a short-term survival advantage with preoperative chemotherapy [5]. Additionally, in the NSABP B-18 trial, more patients in the preoperative group were able to receive lumpectomies, particularly among patients with large tumors. In the preoperative group, the primary tumor response to chemotherapy correlated with outcome, and thus a further advantage of preoperative chemotherapy was the opportunity to observe the primary tumor response, which was not possible in the postoperative group. The advantages of preoperative chemotherapy found in NSABP B18 and similar studies has led to greater use of preoperative or neoadjuvant chemotherapy for women with operable breast cancer, especially those who desire a lumpectomy but have tumors too large at presentation for conservative surgery.

The ability to monitor the primary tumor response is a potentially significant advantage of preoperative chemotherapy. The NSABP B-18 result showing a statistically significant correlation between the primary tumor response and outcome suggest that clinical and pathologic characteristics of the tumor response may provide prognostic information that can be used to guide decisions about continued therapy. There is enormous interest among researchers in identifying such characteristics that might be used to stratify patients in clinically meaningful ways that lead to improvement in survival outcomes. A wide range of measurements can be applied to characterize the tumor response, derived from clinical examination, tissue- or blood-based assays, or in vivo imaging. Immunohistochemical markers of angiogenesis, apoptosis, proliferation, and patterns of gene expression are being actively investigated in neoadjuvant treatment trials to determine if individual or combinations of markers can help identify patients that will go on to have a poor response to treatment.

One breast imaging technique that is being used increasingly because of its high sensitivity to breast cancer and superior ability to demonstrate the extent and distribution of disease is contrast-enhanced MR imaging. Contrast-enhanced MR imaging of the breast is a relatively new diagnostic method that has shown efficacy in the detection of cancer in high-risk women and in cancer staging. The attributes of MR imaging have also led to its

Department of Radiology, University of California, San Francisco, 1 Irving Street, Room AC-109, San Francisco, CA 94143-1290, USA
E-mail address: nola.hylton@radiology.ucsf.edu

1064-9689/06/$ – see front matter © 2006 Elsevier Inc. All rights reserved.
mri.theclinics.com

doi:10.1016/j.mric.2006.09.001

increased use in the evaluation of the preoperative breast and to monitor the primary tumor response to neoadjuvant treatment. It performs better than clinical examination, mammography, or sonography in detecting the extent of cancer after diagnosis to help decide between surgical options or neoadjuvant chemotherapy [6–11]. Contrast-enhanced MR imaging has shown greater accuracy than mammography and sonography for demonstrating the extent of cancer in the breast when compared with histopathology. MR imaging is effective in areas where mammography has limitations, including in dense breast tissue, in the evaluation of lobular carcinoma, and in the presence of ductal carcinoma in situ (DCIS) and multifocal disease. MR imaging is also more effective than clinical examination, mammography, or sonography for documenting the extent of residual disease after chemotherapy, though it is not sufficiently accurate to obviate surgery on the basis of a negative imaging finding.

In addition to its direct clinical use for primary tumor staging, MR imaging in the neoadjuvant treatment setting allows exploration of its potential value in quantifying primary tumor response. The high sensitivity and staging accuracy of MR imaging may yield more accurate classification of objective tumor response using Response Evaluation Criteria in Solid Tumors (RECIST) criteria than clinical examination or mammography. Volumetric measurement of tumor extent, which is made possible with the three-dimensional data generated by MR imaging, could also capture response better than tumor diameter, leading to better stratification of patients into groups with significantly different survival outcomes. In vivo functional measurements of tumor biology using contrast-enhanced MR imaging, diffusion-weighted MR imaging, or MR spectroscopy may yield markers that can be used to predict response to treatment. Functional measurements hold the promise of greater sensitivity for detecting biologic effects of targeted treatments than simple anatomic methods.

MR imaging for assessing residual disease

MR imaging is useful for measuring residual disease after chemotherapy; however, it can miss disease because of reduced signal enhancement due to either decreased contrast uptake as a result of antiangiogenic action of treatment, or partial volume averaging that can occur when the residual disease is distributed diffusely. Several studies have compared contrast-enhanced MR imaging with mammography, sonography, or clinical examination for estimation of residual disease extent following chemotherapy [12–20]. All of these studies were performed in small series of patients, and most reported better correlation of MR imaging with histopathologic residual disease size than the other imaging modalities or clinical examination.

An important treatment outcome that has been found to be associated with higher survival rates is the absence of residual cancer following surgery, or pathologic complete response. It is conceivable that patients with a pathologic complete response could be spared surgery if a noninvasive method could be shown to be accurate in confirming that no residual disease remained following chemotherapy. Schott and colleagues [18] looked specifically at the ability of mammography, sonography and MR imaging to predict pathologic complete response and found comparable accuracy among the imaging methods, but also found that in the case of each of the imaging modalities that residual disease was suggested in one or two of the four cases in which a pathologic complete response was achieved. Other studies of breast MR imaging for assessing response to neoadjuvant chemotherapy have reported both under- and overestimation of residual disease size, with a tendency for MR imaging to underestimate residual disease extent in tumors with significant response [21–27]. In a study by Wasser and colleagues [24], histologic regression was evaluated and scored on the basis of cytopathic effects, reactive changes and tumor cell reduction. The investigators found that the correlation between tumor sizes measured by MR imaging and histopathology was poorer for tumors with regressive changes.

A few studies have reported overestimation of disease extent by MR imaging. Kwong and colleagues [22] compared residual disease estimates by MR imaging with histopathology and found that MR imaging overestimated the extent of disease in four of six patients with pathologic complete response or near complete response. In the same study, MR imaging also overestimated the residual disease size for four axillary lesions that were followed by MR imaging. In the study by Schott and colleagues [18], MR imaging predicted a complete response in only one of four patients showing a pathologic complete response. Partridge and colleagues [13] suggested that the accuracy of breast MR imaging for evaluating residual disease is improved if interpreted relative to the disease extent at baseline and using relaxed enhancement criteria for detecting residual tumor.

MR imaging for monitoring tumor response

If MR imaging is performed before and after neoadjuvant chemotherapy, objective tumor response can be assessed by applying RECIST criteria to the

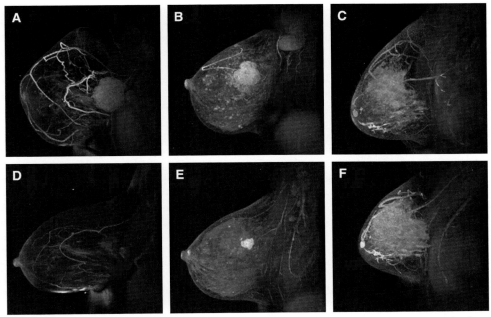

Fig. 1. Prechemotherapy (*top row*) and postchemotherapy (*bottom row*) maximum intensity projection images are shown for three patients demonstrating three different degrees of tumor response: complete tumor response (*A, D*), partial response (*B, E*), and tumor progression on treatment (*C, F*).

primary breast tumor [28]. In Fig. 1, examples of pre- and postchemotherapy maximum intensity projection MR images are shown for three patients having a complete response, partial response and progressive disease on MR imaging. Several studies have compared MR imaging measurements of tumor response with that measured clinically. MR imaging determined rates of complete response, partial response or no response correlated well with response measurements by standard clinical assessment [12,17,19,20].

Other studies have explored MR imaging–measured tumor characteristics evaluated early in treatment for their ability to predict the eventual overall clinical or histopathologic tumor response [29–36]. These studies evaluated size and morphologic measurements by MR imaging as well as functional parameters related to the pharmacokinetics of contrast agent uptake. In a study of 33 patients with advanced breast cancer who underwent serial MR imaging examinations before chemotherapy, after 1 course and following chemotherapy, Cheung and colleagues [32] applied RECIST criteria to MR images to evaluate tumor response and evaluated the early size reduction (ESR) measured after the first course of treatment. ESR was found to correlate with response; patients who had a higher ESR were more likely to have a complete response. Martincich and colleagues [29] measured tumor volume and early contrast uptake in a study of 30 breast

cancer patients receiving neoadjuvant chemotherapy and found that reductions in tumor volume and early contrast uptake after two cycles of treatment were associated with a major histopathologic response, defined as residual disease consisting on either no residual viable cancer cells or only small clusters of dispersed residual cancer cells. In a study of 68 patients with locally advanced breast cancer, Pickles and colleagues [30] found changes in tumor volume and the pharmacokinetic parameters transfer constant (K_{trans}), rate contrast (K_{ep}), and extracellular extravascular space (v_e), measured by MR imaging early in treatment, were significantly different between responding and nonresponding patients, determined on the basis of their final tumor volume reduction. Manton and colleagues [33] applied MR imaging and spectroscopy to measure pharmacokinetic parameters, water apparent diffusion coefficient, fat/water ratio and water T2 before treatment and after the second of six treatment cycles. Pharmacokinetic parameters and apparent diffusion coefficient did not detect an early response, however fat/water ratio and water T2 measurements did correlate with final tumor volume response. Three studies found correlations between the initial morphologic patterns of breast tumors on MR imaging and their likelihood of response to treatment [35–37]. In the study by Esserman and colleagues [36], breast cancers were classified from 1 to 5 according to the degree of tumor containment, where 1 corresponded to unicentric tumors with well-defined boundaries, and 5 corresponded to a septal spreading pattern with ill-defined boundaries (Fig. 2). Morphologic pattern was found to be associated with the tumor response, with 77% of type 1 tumors demonstrating a partial or complete response versus 25% of type 5 tumors. A higher rate of breast conservation was also associated with tumors of type 1 morphologic pattern. Murata and colleagues [35] used a similar classification and found an association between those tumors of the solitary nodular type at presentation and the likelihood of achieving a pathologic complete response with treatment.

Partridge and colleagues [38] reported a study performed at our institution of 62 patients with locally advanced breast cancer who received neoadjuvant chemotherapy, consisting of four cycles of adriamycin and cytoxan (AC). A subset of 12 patients in this group also received 12 weekly cycles of taxane therapy following AC administration. All patients underwent MR imaging examination before chemotherapy and again at the end of chemotherapy. Forty-eight patients also underwent MR imaging after the first cycle of AC. All patients went on to lumpectomy or mastectomy surgery following chemotherapy. The contrast-enhanced MR imaging technique consisted of a three–time point,

high–spatial resolution, three-dimensional method in which one image set was acquired precontrast, and two image sets were acquired after contrast injection. Tumor was defined using an enhancement threshold of 70% in the first postcontrast image on prechemotherapy MR imaging, which was reduced to 40% in the first postcontrast image on postchemotherapy MR imaging. The longest diameter was measured on cross-sectional images, and tumor volume was computed by summing all of the pixels meeting the initial enhancement criteria. Clinical size, residual tumor size on pathology, lymph node status, and MR imaging size measurements were compared for their ability to predict length of recurrence-free survival. Fifty-eight patients were appropriate for analysis and were followed to record occurrences of local or distant disease recurrence or death. The median time to recurrence in the recurrent group (n = 13) was 10 months, and the median follow-up time in the disease-free group (n = 45) was 33 months. In univariate analysis, baseline MR imaging tumor volume, final change in MR imaging tumor volume, baseline MR imaging longest diameter, baseline clinical diameter, residual disease size on pathology, and number of lymph nodes at surgery were all statistically significant ($P<.05$). In subsequent multivariate analysis, only baseline MR imaging volume and

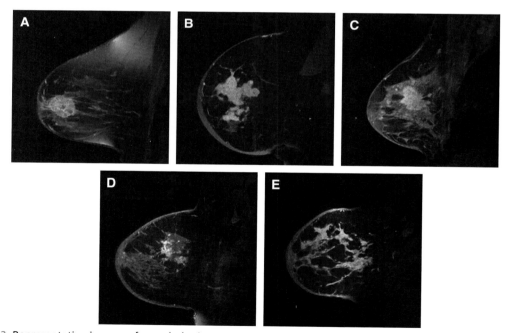

Fig. 2. Representative images of morphologic pattern types 1 through 5 demonstrating degree of tumor containment. (*A*) Pattern 1 corresponds to a unicentric, well-circumscribed tumor. (*B*) Pattern 2 corresponds to a multilobulated tumor with well-circumscribed margin. (*C*) Pattern 3 corresponds to an area enhancement with irregular margins and nodularity. (*D*) Pattern 4 corresponds to an area enhancement with irregular margins and without nodularity. (*E*) Pattern 5 corresponds to enhancement in a dendritic or septal spreading pattern.

final change in volume were found to be significant independent predictors of length of recurrence-free survival. This finding suggests that volume measurements are more accurate at capturing tumor size and change in size as a result of treatment than diameter measurements. The volume measurements in this study were based on a simple threshold, and volume computation was automated, making the measurement technique operator independent and reproducible.

Continuing studies are also evaluating the tumor microvasculature based on the kinetics of contrast agent uptake following injection. In the same group of 67 patients, tumor vascular properties were measured using the signal enhancement ratio (SER) at each pixel meeting the initial signal enhancement threshold. SER was calculated as $(S_1 - S_0)/(S_2 - S_0)$, where S_0 is the precontrast signal intensity, S_1 is the signal intensity of the first postcontrast image, and S_2 is the signal intensity of the second postcontrast image. In addition to measuring longest diameter and volume, breast tumors were characterized at each MR imaging examination by measuring peak values of SER, and and tumor volume fractions by SER range, defined as high SER (SER>1.3), mid-SER (0.9<SER≤1.3), and low SER (SER≤0.9). Tumors were also characterized once at baseline MR imaging according to their morphologic classification. Fig. 3 shows an example for one patient of MR images and SER maps corresponding to the pretreatment, post–AC, and postchemotherapy time points. Quantitative measurements of total tumor volume, peak SER, and high SER are reported for each time point. When SER parameters are considered in combination with clinical and MR imaging size variables, baseline low SER and final change in tumor volume remain significant independent predictors. These results suggest that both both size and kinetic parameters of breast tumors are useful in characterizing tumor response. The American College of Radiology Imaging Network (ACRIN) Trial 6657 is testing the parameters that showed significance in the pilot studies for predicting recurrence-free survival. This trial is being performed in collaboration with the Cancer and Leukemia Group B Trial 150007, which is evaluating tissue and serum-based molecular markers in the same patient cohort.

These studies and others suggest a role for MR imaging in characterizing the response of breast tumors to neoadjuvant chemotherapy to facilitate the assessment of treatment efficacy. Such a method

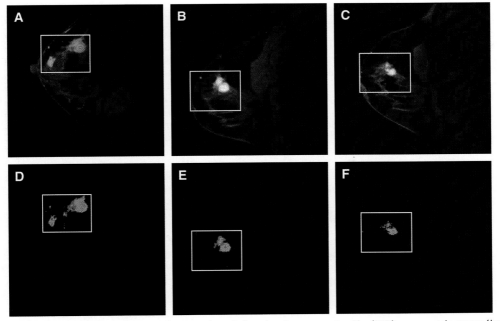

Fig. 3. Contrast-enhanced MR images (*top row*) and signal enhancement ratio (SER) parametric maps (*bottom row*) are shown for a patient with locally advanced breast cancer. Blue, green, and red color coding corresponds to low (SER<0.9), moderate (0.9≤SER≤1.1), and high (SER>1.1) values, respectively. (*A, D*) Precontrast (baseline) MR images. (*B, E*) Chemotherapy images after one cycle. (*C, F*) Postchemotherapy images. Baseline: volume (cm³), 5.2; hotspot SER, 2.0; high SER volume (cm³), 0.52; high SER volume fraction (%), 10. After one cycle: volume (cm³), 2.1; hotspot SER, 1.3; high SER volume (cm³), 0.04; high SER volume fraction (%), 2. After 4 cycles: volume (cm³), 1.4; hotspot SER, 1.5; high SER volume (cm³), 0.19; high SER volume fraction (%), 13.

that can be used noninvasively and repeatedly to evaluate patients during treatment is of particular importance as more new and promising therapeutic agents become available. Imaging techniques that quantitatively assess response, both morphologically and functionally, are being integrated into oncologic clinical trials to test their ability to measure the effects of treatment and to explore the value of imaging measurements for predicting treatment benefit. These trials provide clinical and histopathologic correlates that are needed to properly assess the efficacy of the imaging techniques. The data provided by these clinical trials will hopefully help to determine the most effective imaging approaches for monitoring patients during treatment.

References

[1] Fisher B, Bryant J, Wolmark N, et al. Effect of pre-operative chemotherapy on the outcome of women with operable breast cancer. J Clin Oncol 1998;16:2672–85.

[2] Wolmark N, Wang J, Mamounas E, et al. Preoperative chemotherapy in patients with operable breast cancer: nine-year results from National Surgical Adjuvant Breast and Bowel Project B-18. J Natl Cancer Inst Monogr 2001;96–102.

[3] Makris A, Powles TJ, Ashley SE, et al. A reduction in the requirements for mastectomy in a randomized trial of neoadjuvant chemoendocrine therapy in primary breast cancer. Ann Oncol 1998; 9:1179–84.

[4] Mauriac L, MacGrogan G, Avril A, et al. Neoadjuvant chemotherapy for operable breast carcinoma larger than 3 cm: a unicentre randomized trial with a 124-month median follow-up. Institut Bergonie Bordeaux Groupe Sein (IBBGS). Ann Oncol 1999;10:47–52.

[5] Broet P, Scholl SM, de la Rochefordiere A, et al. Short and long-term effects on survival in breast cancer patients treated by primary chemotherapy: an updated analysis of a randomized trial. Breast Cancer Res Treat 1999;58:151–6.

[6] Mumtaz H, Hall-Craggs MA, Davidson T, et al. Staging of symptomatic primary breast cancer with MR imaging. AJR Am J Roentgenol 1997; 169:417–24.

[7] Van Goethem M, Schelfout K, Dijckmans L, et al. MR mammography in the pre-operative staging of breast cancer in patients with dense breast tissue: comparison with mammography and ultrasound. Eur Radiol 2004;14:809–16.

[8] Esserman L, Hylton N, Yassa L, et al. Utility of magnetic resonance imaging in the management of breast cancer: evidence for improved preoperative staging. J Clin Oncol 1999;17:110–9.

[9] Kramer S, Schulz-Wendtland R, Hagedorn K, et al. Magnetic resonance imaging and its role in the diagnosis of multicentric breast cancer. Anticancer Res 1998;18:2163–4.

[10] Boetes C, Mus RD, Holland R, et al. Breast tumors: comparative accuracy of MR imaging relative to mammography and US for demonstrating extent. Radiology 1995;197:743–7.

[11] Davis PL, Staiger MJ, Harris KB, et al. Breast cancer measurements with magnetic resonance imaging, ultrasonography, and mammography. Breast Cancer Res Treat 1996;37:1–9.

[12] Drew PJ, Kerin MJ, Mahapatra T, et al. Evaluation of response to neoadjuvant chemoradiotherapy for locally advanced breast cancer with dynamic contrast-enhanced MRI of the breast. Eur J Surg Oncol 2001;27:617–20.

[13] Partridge SC, Gibbs JE, Lu Y, et al. Accuracy of MR imaging for revealing residual breast cancer in patients who have undergone neoadjuvant chemotherapy. AJR Am J Roentgenol 2002;179:1193–9.

[14] Londero V, Bazzocchi M, Del Frate C, et al. Locally advanced breast cancer: comparison of mammography, sonography and MR imaging in evaluation of residual disease in women receiving neoadjuvant chemotherapy. Eur Radiol 2004;14:1371–9.

[15] Yeh E, Slanetz P, Kopans DB, et al. Prospective comparison of mammography, sonography, and MRI in patients undergoing neoadjuvant chemotherapy for palpable breast cancer. AJR Am J Roentgenol 2005;184:868–77.

[16] Montemurro F, Martincich L, De Rosa G, et al. Dynamic contrast-enhanced MRI and sonography in patients receiving primary chemotherapy for breast cancer. Eur Radiol 2005;15:1224–33.

[17] Akazawa K, Tamaki Y, Taguchi T, et al. Preoperative evaluation of residual tumor extent by three-dimensional magnetic resonance imaging in breast cancer patients treated with neoadjuvant chemotherapy. Breast J 2006;12:130–7.

[18] Schott AF, Roubidoux MA, Helvie MA, et al. Clinical and radiologic assessments to predict breast cancer pathologic complete response to neoadjuvant chemotherapy. Breast Cancer Res Treat 2005;92:231–8.

[19] Abraham DC, Jones RC, Jones SE, et al. Evaluation of neoadjuvant chemotherapeutic response of locally advanced breast cancer by magnetic resonance imaging. Cancer 1996;78:91–100.

[20] Balu-Maestro C, Chapellier C, Bleuse A, et al. Imaging in evaluation of response to neoadjuvant breast cancer treatment benefits of MRI. Breast Cancer Res Treat 2002;72:145–52.

[21] Weatherall PT, Evans GF, Metzger GJ, et al. MRI vs. histologic measurement of breast cancer following chemotherapy: comparison with x-ray mammography and palpation. J Magn Reson Imaging 2001;13:868–75.

[22] Kwong MS, Chung GG, Horvath LJ, et al. Postchemotherapy MRI overestimates residual disease compared with histopathology in responders to neoadjuvant therapy for locally advanced breast cancer. Cancer J 2006;12:212–21.

[23] Rieber A, Brambs HJ, Gabelmann A, et al. Breast MRI for monitoring response of primary breast

cancer to neo-adjuvant chemotherapy. Eur Radiol 2002;12:1711–9.

[24] Wasser K, Sinn HP, Fink C, et al. Accuracy of tumor size measurement in breast cancer using MRI is influenced by histological regression induced by neoadjuvant chemotherapy. Eur Radiol 2003;13:1213–23.

[25] Denis F, Desbiez-Bourcier AV, Chapiron C, et al. Contrast enhanced magnetic resonance imaging underestimates residual disease following neoadjuvant docetaxel based chemotherapy for breast cancer. Eur J Surg Oncol 2004;30:1069–76.

[26] Warren RM, Bobrow LG, Earl HM, et al. Can breast MRI help in the management of women with breast cancer treated by neoadjuvant chemotherapy? Br J Cancer 2004;90:1349–60.

[27] Rosen EL, Blackwell KL, Baker JA, et al. Accuracy of MRI in the detection of residual breast cancer after neoadjuvant chemotherapy. AJR Am J Roentgenol 2003;181:1275–82.

[28] Therasse P, Arbuck SG, Eisenhauer EA, et al. New guidelines to evaluate the response to treatment in solid tumors. European Organization for Research and Treatment of Cancer, National Cancer Institute of the United States, National Cancer Institute of Canada. J Natl Cancer Inst 2000;92:205–16.

[29] Martincich L, Montemurro F, De Rosa G, et al. Monitoring response to primary chemotherapy in breast cancer using dynamic contrast-enhanced magnetic resonance imaging. Breast Cancer Res Treat 2004;83:67–76.

[30] Pickles MD, Lowry M, Manton DJ, et al. Role of dynamic contrast enhanced MRI in monitoring early response of locally advanced breast cancer to neoadjuvant chemotherapy. Breast Cancer Res Treat 2005;91:1–10.

[31] Padhani AR, Hayes C, Assersohn L, et al. Prediction of clinicopathologic response of breast cancer to primary chemotherapy at contrast-enhanced MR imaging: initial clinical results. Radiology 2006;239:361–74.

[32] Cheung YC, Chen SC, Su MY, et al. Monitoring the size and response of locally advanced breast cancers to neoadjuvant chemotherapy (weekly paclitaxel and epirubicin) with serial enhanced MRI. Breast Cancer Res Treat 2003;78:51–8.

[33] Manton DJ, Chaturvedi A, Hubbard A, et al. Neoadjuvant chemotherapy in breast cancer: early response prediction with quantitative MR imaging and spectroscopy. Br J Cancer 2006;94:427–35.

[34] Wasser K, Klein SK, Fink C, et al. Evaluation of neoadjuvant chemotherapeutic response of breast cancer using dynamic MRI with high temporal resolution. Eur Radiol 2003;13:80–7.

[35] Murata Y, Ogawa Y, Yoshida S, et al. Utility of initial MRI for predicting extent of residual disease after neoadjuvant chemotherapy: analysis of 70 breast cancer patients. Oncol Rep 2004;12:1257–62.

[36] Esserman L, Kaplan E, Partridge S, et al. MRI phenotype is associated with response to doxorubicin and cyclophosphamide neoadjuvant chemotherapy in stage III breast cancer. Ann Surg Oncol 2001;8:549–59.

[37] Martincich L, Montemurro F, Cirillo S, et al. Role of magnetic resonance imaging in the prediction of tumor response in patients with locally advanced breast cancer receiving neoadjuvant chemo-therapy. Radiol Med (Torino) 2003;106:51–8.

[38] Partridge SC, Gibbs JE, Lu Y, et al. MRI measurements of breast tumor volume predict response to neoadjuvant chemotherapy and recurrence-free survival. AJR Am J Roentgenol 2005;184:1774–81.

MAGNETIC
RESONANCE
IMAGING CLINICS

Magn Reson Imaging Clin N Am 14 (2006) 391–402

MR Imaging for Surveillance of Women at High Familial Risk for Breast Cancer

Christiane K. Kuhl, MD

- Who is at increased risk for breast cancer?
- Some basic facts regarding familial or hereditary breast cancer
- What are the current options regarding prevention?
- Specific aspects regarding the design of a surveillance program for women with familial breast cancer
  Who should be offered intensified surveillance?

At which age should one start with surveillance? Which interval is appropriate?
What other factors may influence the design of a surveillance program?
- Efficacy of different breast imaging modalities for early diagnosis of familial or hereditary breast cancer
- References

Who is at increased risk for breast cancer?

The average lifetime risk for breast cancer amounts to approximately 10% to 12% in women in the Western world [1]. A variety of conditions are associated with a cumulative risk, however, that may go far beyond this average. An increased risk can be expected in women with a prior history of breast cancer or in patients who have had a tissue diagnosis of borderline biologic behavior, such as atypical ductal hyperplasia (ADH) or lobular carcinoma in situ (LCIS). It can also be expected in patients who have undergone mediastinal irradiation for Hodgkin's disease, for example. Finally, a familial clustering of breast or ovarian cancer, particularly in cases with early onset, goes along with an increased lifetime risk. Cancers arising in this latter group are usually referred to as "familial" or "hereditary" breast cancers. The distinction between familial and hereditary breast cancer can be difficult in the individual case. In general, *familial cancer* is a descriptive term that indicates an increased incidence of breast cancer on the same side of a family. The term *hereditary breast cancer* suggests that a specific germline mutation in a breast cancer susceptibility gene is passed on in the family and has been identified by mutational analysis or is suspected on the basis of pedigree analysis revealing a specific (eg, autosomal dominant) inheritance pattern [2].

Some basic facts regarding familial or hereditary breast cancer

Approximately 10% of the new breast cancers diagnosed each year are attributable to hereditary breast cancer. In addition, family history is in itself one of the most important risk factors for sporadic breast cancer; by numbers, this is a much larger group than breast cancer that arises because of a single site-specific mutation.

Department of Radiology, University of Bonn, Sigmund-Freud-Strasse 25, D-53105 Bonn, Germany
E-mail address: kuhl@uni-bonn.de

1064-9689/06/$ – see front matter © 2006 Elsevier Inc. All rights reserved.
mri.theclinics.com

doi:10.1016/j.mric.2006.07.003

The breast and ovarian cancer susceptibility genes identified thus far, BRCA1 and BRCA2, account for approximately 50% of the actual hereditary breast cancer cases; the remaining half of hereditary cancers seem to be caused by other as yet unidentified genes ("BRCAX"). Most cancers in this second half are probably be attributable to a variety of further predisposing, probably low-penetrance, genes that have not been identified to date [3–6]. Women with a documented pathogenic BRCA mutation face a substantially increased lifetime risk for breast and ovarian cancer. The lifetime risk for breast cancer accumulates to 60% to 85% for carriers of the BRCA1 and BRCA2 mutations, respectively [7,8]. For carriers of BRCA1 and BRCA2, the average age at first diagnosis of breast cancer is younger than that observed in women with sporadic breast cancer. According to recent data, approximately 50% of such patients already had breast cancer by the age of 50 years. In BRCA1 mutation carriers, the risk increases from the age of 25 years onward continuously to peak in the group between 45 and 49 years of age (with annual incidence rates of >4%) and decays thereafter. Also, and again in contrast to women with sporadic breast cancer, women with a BRCA mutation face a high risk of developing a second primary breast cancer, which has been estimated to be as high as 60%.

Breast cancers arising in mutation carriers tend to exhibit adverse histopathologic features that are indicative of aggressive biologic behavior; with respect to sporadic breast cancers, they exhibit high proliferation rates, are more likely to show high nuclear grading and medullar or atypical-medullar differentiation, and are more often receptor-negative [9–12].

What are the current options regarding prevention?

There are several options available for the management of (or rather the care for) women with suspected or proved hereditary breast cancer [13–16]. Primary prevention aims at reducing the incidence of familial breast cancer in women at high risk. It can be achieved by risk-reducing surgical interventions, such as prophylactic mastectomy or salpingo-oophorectomy, and (with less consistent results) possibly also by antihormonal treatment with tamoxifen, for example, for chemoprevention.

Preventive salpingo-oophorectomy has been shown to reduce the risk of subsequent breast cancer by approximately 30%. In addition, it does, of course, reduce the risk of ovarian cancer. The latter is important because there are virtually no effective imaging strategies for early diagnosis of ovarian cancer. Accordingly, preventive oophorectomy serves two purposes at the same time and is recommended in women after child-bearing age.

Although there is substantial evidence to support preventive oophorectomy, preventive mastectomy is usually not propagated as a first-line choice for the management of women with familial breast cancer. Although in documented mutation carriers, the lifetime risk accumulates to 80%, this means that some 20% of women never develop breast cancer. The situation is even more difficult for women without an identifiable mutation, in whom it may be difficult to predict the actual lifetime risk. In the absence of a detectable pathogenic mutation, family history is used to corroborate risk prediction, a technique that is increasingly difficult to apply with the increasing number of small single-child families. The perceived mutilating effects of mastectomy, together with the difficulty in predicting the outcome in individual cases, make the decision for surgical prevention difficult for most women. Still, it is important to note that preventive mastectomy has been demonstrated to be efficient in that it significantly reduces the incidence of breast cancer [17–20].

Secondary prevention (ie, intensified surveillance) aims at the earliest possible diagnosis of familial breast cancer at a prognostically favorable stage. The underlying assumption is that the same correlation exists between stage at diagnosis and outcome (eg, morbidity, mortality) as has been demonstrated for sporadic breast cancer. This, however, has not been proven to date, and there is evidence to suggest that the correlation between stage at diagnosis and ultimate prognosis may not be as clear for women with hereditary breast cancer as it is for women with sporadic disease [21].

Specific aspects regarding the design of a surveillance program for women with familial breast cancer

There are several features of familial breast cancer that should affect the design of any given surveillance protocol.

Who should be offered intensified surveillance?

The identification of women whose risk for breast cancer is increased to an extent that justifies genetic testing and participation in an intensified surveillance program should be the task of a specialized geneticist. Although there are computer programs available that help with the calculation of lifetime risk, the results have to be interpreted with great care and have to be adequately communicated to the person who seeks this advice. Many women with a family history of breast cancer overestimate their own risk and may tend to self-refer for screening studies. More often than not, these women can be reassured after qualified genetic counseling, because the perceived risk is higher than the actual calculated lifetime risk.

For the time being, only mutations in the BRCA1 and BRCA2 genes are amenable to genetic testing. Because approximately half of the actual hereditary breast cancers (and many of the familial breast cancers) are not associated with BRCA1 or BRCA2, however, a positive test result should not be required as an inclusion criterion for entry in an intensified surveillance program. Instead, women without a documented mutation (or women who refuse to undergo mutational analysis) should be included provided that the personal or family history yields a calculated lifetime risk that exceeds a certain threshold. Usually, the cutoff is set at a lifetime risk of 20% or greater. A negative test result is not predictive and may not be used to dismiss an individual from intensified surveillance. This is true, with the exception of the following situation: if an individual tests negative for a specific mutation that has been identified in the index patient, this can be used confidently to classify this individual as having no increased risk but an average risk.

Because of the high risk of second primary breast cancers, intensified surveillance should also be offered to women who were already diagnosed with familial or hereditary breast cancer. In these individuals, the probability of a second primary breast cancer developing is higher than the probability of the first primary breast cancer recurring. Accordingly, surveillance serves two purposes: follow-up of the symptomatic breast and screening of the contralateral side.

At which age should one start with surveillance? Which interval is appropriate?

Because of the early onset of the disease, screening of women with suspected hereditary breast cancer should start at a substantially earlier age than what is recommended for the general population and should be continued even after an individual has been diagnosed with breast cancer. Virtually all existing guidelines recommend to start screening at the age of 30 years (at the latest), or 5 years before the youngest family member with the disease. This has an immediate impact on the accuracy of diagnostic imaging, because women at the age of 30 years have much denser fibroglandular tissue than the usual case of a woman 50 years of age or older at average risk who undergoes regular screening. The probability is high that the higher parenchymal density may cause equivocal mammographic findings more often, which may require clarification by short-term mammographic follow-up, additional

mammographic views, or biopsy. It is well established [22] that the diagnostic accuracy of mammography (positive predictive value [PPV] regarding sensitivity as well as specificity) is statistically significantly reduced in women in the age group of 40 through 49 years because of their, on average, denser parenchymal patterns compared with women aged 50 years and older. Even more diagnostic difficulties can be predicted to occur in women younger than 40 years of age.

Because of the relative biologic aggressiveness (rapid proliferation rates) of familial breast cancer, the lead time (ie, the time during which a cancer can be diagnosed by imaging studies in its subclinical stage) is short. Accordingly, screening intervals have to be kept short compared with those in women at average risk. There are no data available to date that would systematically evaluate the impact of different screening intervals on cancer yield and stage at diagnosis or number of interval cancers. In the absence of available data, most existing protocols recommend annual screening intervals for mammography (and MR imaging, if at all mentioned); ultrasound, if integrated, is usually recommended semiannually. This recommendation is given not to acknowledge the superior diagnostic value of breast ultrasound compared with mammography or MR imaging but because breast ultrasound is relatively inexpensive, broadly available, and does not use ionizing radiation; as such, it seems suitable for use as an interim imaging modality between regular screening rounds.

In view of the need for early onset of screening, the short screening intervals, and the high probability at which additional mammographic views are required for problem solving, it is of interest that BRCA-related gene products have been implicated in cell cycle regeneration and DNA repair [23–25]. In particular, the products of the intact BRCA1 gene locus seem to play a role in the repair of DNA double-strand breaks (ie, a mutation that is typically caused by ionizing radiation). Although the in vivo effects of the BRCA malfunction are still unclear and are subject to current research, to date and until proven otherwise, it seems prudent to assume an increased radiosensitivity in women with a pathogenic BRCA mutation. Although even in the worst case, the attributable risk is still small compared with the natural lifetime risk in mutation carriers, this fact should prompt health care providers to an even more careful and judicious use of ionizing radiation in this specific subset of women. With the current guidelines for intensified surveillance, there is no doubt that women with a documented or possible mutation are, in fact, exposed to a substantially higher cumulative lifetime dose than women at average risk. The possible biologic effects of this "intensified mammographic screening" are unknown and have to be carefully evaluated and weighed against the (limited) benefit of mammographic screening in mutation carriers.

In the past, the possibly increased radiosensitivity of mutation carriers has been one of the major reasons to discourage the use of breast-conserving treatment in women who were diagnosed with operable familial breast cancer, because the late sequelae of radiation therapy were unknown. Recent outcome results suggest, however, that mutation carriers who underwent radiation therapy exhibit a reduced risk of local recurrence compared with age- and stage-matched patients with sporadic breast cancer. This is interpreted as being attributable to the increased radiosensitivity of the BRCA-associated breast cancers themselves, which turns out to be beneficial. Accordingly, to date, breast conservation is a viable option for women with early-stage familial breast cancer [26–31].

What other factors may influence the design of a surveillance program?

In addition to the diagnostic difficulties that are attributable to the increased density of the fibroglandular tissue of young women at high risk, there is another reason why familial breast cancer may be difficult to diagnose. It has been shown that familial breast cancers—not only those with medullar differentiation but the "regular" duct invasive cancers—frequently exhibit morphologic features that are usually indicative of benign lesions. BRCA1-associated cancers tend to exhibit "pushing" well-circumscribed margins and a roundish or oval configuration at mammography. In breast ultrasound, the lesions exhibit a homogeneous internal architecture with low echogenicity; in short, these cancers may be indistinguishable from benign fibroadenomas or even cysts on mammographic and ultrasound imaging studies (Fig. 1) [26,32]. Accordingly, in addition to the difficulties caused by the high parenchymal density, the misleadingly benign imaging features of familial breast cancers contribute to the reduced diagnostic accuracy of mammography (also of breast ultrasound) in mutation carriers.

Efficacy of different breast imaging modalities for early diagnosis of familial or hereditary breast cancer

A number of guidelines have been published on the appropriate clinical management of women at calculated high genetic risk. Most of these programs, however, have been based on expert opinion alone and not on data of prospective clinical trials.

Still, virtually all existing guidelines and programs recommend to have women at high genetic risk undergo mammographic screening on an annual basis, starting at the age of 30 years (at the latest), usually accompanied by clinical breast examination (CBE) or breast self-examination (BSE).

This is in spite of the fact that the experiences reported for mammographic screening in women at increased genetic risk have indeed been discouraging [33–36]. The overall sensitivity of mammographic screening is unacceptably low. The rate of interval cancers (ie, the number of individuals in whom early diagnosis failed) has been reported to be as high as 36% to 56% with mammographic screening. This means that mammographic screening did not allow an early diagnosis in more than one third or even up to one half of the women who develop breast cancer. This sobering data prompted a search for other nonmammographic breast imaging techniques, namely, breast ultrasound and MR imaging. Nuclear medicine breast imaging techniques like scintimammography and positron emission tomography (PET) have not been systematically evaluated in women at increased risk for breast cancer. Based on the results in women with sporadic breast cancer, there is no reason to assume that PET or single photon emission computed tomography (SPECT) is suitable for this purpose.

The first data on multimodality screening in women at increased genetic risk were published by our institution in 2000 [32]. A total 192 women who, based on genetic testing or family history, were considered or proven to be carriers of a breast cancer susceptibility gene, underwent systematic screening with mammography, ultrasound, and breast MR imaging for at least 2 years. These preliminary results showed that with MR imaging, the sensitivity for familial breast cancer was more than doubled compared with mammography and even for the combined use of mammography and breast ultrasound.

It has become increasingly clear that the denser fibroglandular tissue in the young women screened was only part of the problem. In addition, diagnostic interpretation errors are caused by the atypical (benign) imaging features of BRCA1-associated breast cancer. Finally, the data documented that the increased sensitivity afforded by MR imaging was not achieved at the expense of specificity. Specificity and PPV (ie, fraction of correct biopsy recommendations or rate of true-positive versus false-positive diagnoses) of breast MR imaging in our hands were comparable to those achieved with mammography and higher by far than those achieved with breast ultrasound.

Meanwhile, a number of prospective clinical trials that aim at comparing the respective cancer yield of other nonmammographic imaging modalities

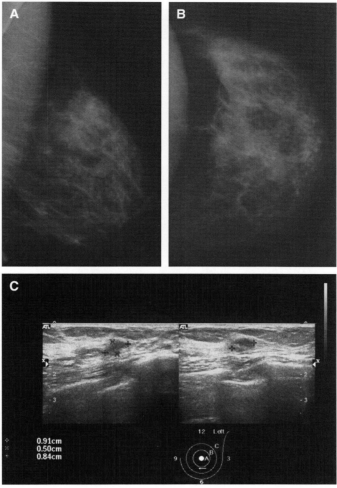

Fig. 1. A 37-year-old patient with a history of breast cancer on her left at the age of 35 years. She was treated with breast conservation, with routine follow-up and no clinical findings. (*A,B*) Mammogram (medio-lateral oblique (MLO) and cranio-caudal (CC) views, left breast). (*C*) Screening breast ultrasound. (*D–L*) Screening breast MR imaging. Precontrast T1-weighted image of the dynamic series (*D*), early postcontrast T1-weighted image of the dynamic series (*E*), early postcontrast subtracted image (*F*), corresponding section of the T2-weighted turbo spin echo (TSE) pulse sequence (without fat suppression) (*G*), enlarged view of early postcontrast T1-weighted image of the dynamic series (*H*), enlarged view of the late postcontrast subtracted image (*I*), enlarged view of corresponding section of the T2-weighted TSE pulse sequence (without fat suppression) (*J*), and time signal intensity curve of the enhancing mass (*K*). The mammogram appears benign with some architectural distortions that were unchanged compared with previous films and interpreted as scar after breast-conserving surgery and radiation therapy. At screening ultrasound, an oval mass was identified with an orientation parallel to the chest wall and Cooper's ligaments. The differential diagnosis ranged between a collapsed cyst, fibroadenoma, and well-defined breast cancer. Breast MR imaging confirmed the presence of a roundish mass with smooth borders [note that the borders are, in fact, microlobulated in the T2-weighted TSE image in (*G*)]. There is strong and early enhancement, followed by wash-out [visible in (*I*) and in the time signal intensity curve in (*K*)], which is not suggestive of fibroadenoma. In addition, the internal architecture of the lesion does not exhibit septations but appears homogeneous. In a T2-weighted TSE image, the mass appears dark, again not suggestive of myxoid fibroadenoma. The MR imaging scan was called suspicious (Breast Imaging and Reporting Data System [BI-RADS] 5) for cancer. Lobular invasive cancer was identified at ultrasound-guided biopsy.

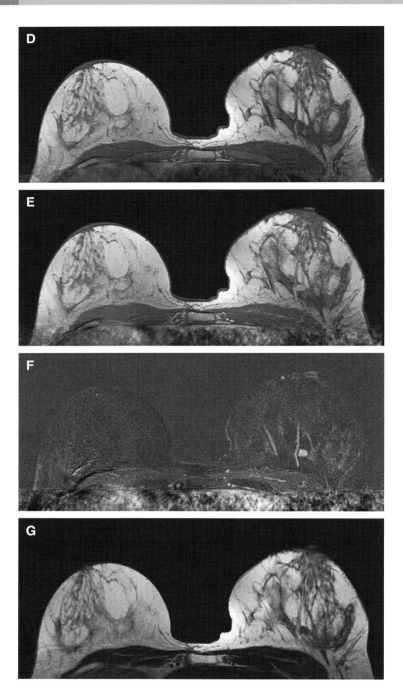

Fig. 1 (continued)

compared with mammographic screening alone have been reported or are underway (Table 1) [32,37–43]. Virtually all trials that have been reported or that are currently recruiting offered (or offer) annual mammographic screening with annual MR imaging; a smaller fraction of trials also investigate the use of breast ultrasound in young high-risk women. The results of these trials are surprisingly concordant in that they confirm that breast MR imaging offers a substantially increased sensitivity for diagnosing familial breast cancer. The data are less concordant regarding the specificity and PPV of MR imaging and the role of mammographic screening.

A higher rate of false-positive diagnoses (ie, lower specificity and PPV) for MR imaging compared with

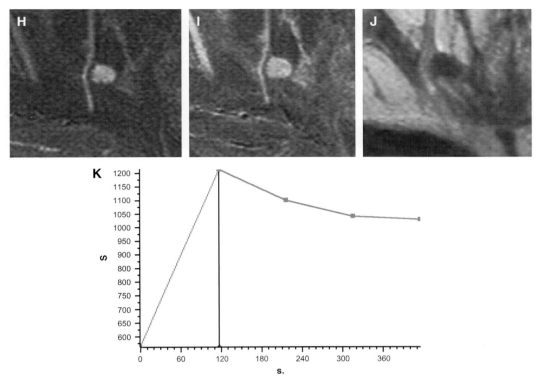

Fig. 1 (continued)

mammography has been reported in several of the studies [38–40,42]. The recent study published by Warner and colleagues [39] provides a good explanation for this. Whereas the rate of false-positive biopsy calls of MR imaging was high in the first year (ie, at the beginning of the breast MR imaging screening project), it decreased from year to year to reach the same level as mammography after 4 years into the program, when mammography and MR imaging exhibited equivalent PPVs. This observation (as well as the results from our trial [32]) suggests that a limited PPV (ie, a high rate of false-positive calls) is not a technique-inherent feature of breast MR imaging. Rather, this is attributable to a limited experience of radiologists with this technique specifically in a screening setting and even more so regarding screening women aged 30 to 39 years, in whom hormonal stimulation of the normal fibroglandular tissue may mimic all sorts of benign and malignant breast lesions (Fig. 2).

It is well established that the accuracy of any diagnostic imaging modality depends heavily on the personal experience of the interpreting radiologist. Specifically regarding mammographic screening, this has led to the recommendation to require a certain number of mammograms to be read each year by radiologists who wish to participate in screening (the current European guidelines require that a minimum of 5000 mammograms be read each year by each radiologist). There is no reason to assume that reading screening breast MR imaging or breast ultrasound scans would require less expertise with these imaging modalities, respectively. Although in the United States alone, more than 40,000,000 screening mammograms are read each year, the total number of breast MR imaging studies is estimated to range between 6000 and 9000 per year until 2002 and up to 22,000 in 2004. This wide gap between the presumed average expertise in reading mammograms compared with the respective expertise in reading breast MR imaging studies is probably the single most important contributor to the reported high rate of false-positive biopsy recommendations made with breast MR imaging. One may even speculate that if mammograms were read with the same level of expertise that the average breast MR imaging study is read, the PPV (rate of false-positive biopsy recommendations) of mammographic screening would, in turn, be inappropriately high. Based on the study by Warner and colleagues [38,39] or the new results from our site, there is evidence to suggest that with increasing practical experience, screening MR imaging has not only an equivalent but, in fact, a higher PPV compared with mammographic or ultrasound screening. So, it seems that the allegedly

Table 1: Comparison of nonmammographic imaging compared with mammographic screening

Study	No. individuals	No. breast cancers	MR imaging		Mammography	
			Sensitivity (%)	Specificity (%)	Sensitivity (%)	Specificity (%)
Kuhl et al, 2000 [32]	192	12	100	95	33	93
Tilanus-Linthorst et al, 2002 [44]	109	3	100	94	0	NA
Stoutjesdijk et al, 2001 [37]	179	14	100	93	42	96
Warner et al, 2001 [38]	196	7	100	91	28	99.5
Podo et al, 2002 [41]	105	8	100	99	12	100
Trecate et al, 2003 [43]	24	4	100	NA	0	NA
Kuhl et al, 2003 [48]	462	51	96	95	43	94
Kriege et al, 2004 [40]	1909	45	80	90	33	95
Warner et al, 2004 [39]	236	22	77	95	36	99
Leach et al, 2005 [47]	649	35	77	81	40	93
Kuhl et al, 2005 [45]	618	12	83	NA	42	NA
Kuhl et al, 2005 [46]	529	43	91	97	33	97

Abbreviation: NA, not applicable.

high false-positive rate of breast MR imaging is, at the same time, the cause and effect of the continued underuse of this technique, thus perpetuating the current situation.

Because hormonal stimulation is a notorious cause of benign contrast enhancement in premenopausal women, our approach to reduce false-positive biopsy recommendations is as follows. If, in a premenopausal woman who is screened, a lesion is identified on MR imaging that exhibits non–mass-like enhancement and has no clinical correlate (eg, palpable lump) and no correlate on second-look ultrasound, we would recommend a follow-up breast MR imaging study in 3 months (in documented mutation carriers or those with a calculated lifetime risk >40%) or in 6 months (other). The second-look ultrasound should be performed by a radiologist who is able to interpret MR imaging studies to ensure that the targeted ultrasound is done at the site of the MR imaging–detected abnormality. If a suspicious abnormality is identified at this second-look ultrasound, an ultrasound-guided core biopsy is performed. If the lesion appears benign on ultrasound, further management is decided based on the MR imaging appearance.

Settling diagnostic problems by recommending follow-up studies in high-risk women is problematic because of the high growth rates of BRCA-associated breast cancers. Therefore, a recommendation to follow up a lesion must be given with caution and should be considered only if all the previously mentioned criteria are fulfilled. A follow-up period of 6 months cannot be considered short term in BRCA mutation carriers or women with equivalent lifetime risk. BRCA-associated breast cancer has been shown to grow extremely fast, such that within

6 months, breast cancer can achieve a considerable size. Therefore, short-term follow-up intervals should be kept at approximately 3 months. This is also justifiable because the main differential diagnosis for non–mass-like enhancement (ie, hormonal stimulation) exhibits a fast fluctuation from one menstrual period to the next, such that there is reason to assume that the enhancing area has resolved after three menstrual cycles (see Fig. 2).

A high rate of false-positive and false-negative diagnoses may also be anticipated if the diagnostic criteria that are used are not updated to current standards. For example, it is well established that the diagnosis of intraductal cancer may not be based on the assessment of enhancement kinetics. If a purely dynamic acquisition is used and only kinetic criteria are applied (ie, naming everything suspicious that exhibits early and strong enhancement, irrespective of distribution and internal architecture), it can be predicted that this approach is not going to capable of identifying ductal carcinoma in situ (DCIS). In fact, a Dutch study [40] showed a relatively high percentage of breast cancers that were false-negative on MR imaging but were diagnosed only because of mammographic abnormalities. This high rate of false-negative MR imaging was not observed in the other trials. Most negative MR imaging cases were attributable to DCIS that went undetected by MR imaging.

To date, however, this means that mammography must still be considered indispensable in women at high genetic risk. Whether or not a compromise may be set by reducing the number of mammographic views per examination, for example, has to be investigated by further studies.

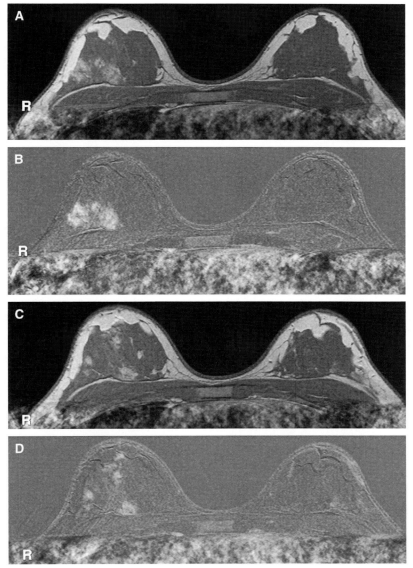

Fig. 2. A 32-year-old woman at high familial risk for breast cancer underwent intensified surveillance. (*A,B*) Images from the regular screening round in March 2002. (*C,D*) Images from a short-term follow-up study that was done 3 months later in June 2002. First postcontrast nonsubtracted image of the dynamic series obtained in March 2002 (*A*), corresponding subtracted image (*B*), postcontrast nonsubtracted image of the dynamic series in June 2002 (*C*), and corresponding subtracted image (*D*). Note the asymmetric non–mass-like regional enhancement that occurs in the prepectoral (posterior) region of the upper outer quadrant of the right breast. No clinical correlate existed. The mammogram was normal, as was the second-look ultrasound scan. Possible hormonal stimulation was suspected, and the patient was scheduled for short-term follow-up. At this follow-up study, the enhancement in the prepectoral region had resolved and other enhancing areas had newly appeared. A second-look ultrasound scan did not reveal any abnormalities at the site of the MR imaging–detectable enhancement. Hormonal stimulation was diagnosed, and the patient was put back to regular screening intervals. Follow-up for more than 3 years has been uneventful.

Without exception, all trials that are underway or have been reported are so-called "observational cohort studies." No randomized trials (with women being randomized into different treatment arms [ie, different screening protocols consisting of single or multimodality screening examinations]) have been reported to date, and no such trial is underway. It is difficult to initiate anything close to the huge population-based mammographic screening trials that were performed in the 1970s. This is not only because of the fact that breast MR imaging is not available on a mass screening level; the number of women who belong to the "high-risk" category is relatively small, and the care of these women is usually not provided on a community-based level but is reserved to specialized centers anyway. The reason is because breast cancer awareness is high at the present time, particularly among families with several affected individuals. Probably more so than in the past, women now tend to seek independent information resources (eg, via the media or the Internet). Based on the limited evidence that exists today on the use of MR imaging for screening familial breast cancer, it is difficult to withhold MR imaging from women at increased risk, particularly if this is done for study purposes alone. Accordingly, it is likely to be increasingly difficult to set up a randomized screening trial that would be needed to investigate the efficacy of intensified screening in terms of mortality.

In conclusion, the current data suggest that MR imaging should be considered an integral part of the surveillance protocol of women at high genetic risk. The role of mammography in this specific group of women needs to be evaluated by further clinical trials.

It is important to note that the data available to date do not allow an outcome analysis. This is in contrast to preventive mastectomy, for which data are available that support its use as a risk-reducing strategy. Whether or not intensified surveillance is effective in terms of reducing morbidity and mortality remains to be seen, however. This lack of evidence must be communicated to individuals at increased genetic risk, and this lack of proven outcome needs to be considered in the decision-making process for appropriate management strategies in each case.

References

[1] Ries LAG, Harkins D, Krapcho M, et al. SEER cancer statistics review 1975–2003. National Cancer Institute, Bethesda, MD. Available at: http://seer.cancer.gov/csr/1975_2003.

[2] Lynch HT, Albano WA, Danes BS, et al. Genetic predisposition to breast cancer. Cancer 1984; 53:612–22.

[3] Miki Y, Swensen J, Shattuck-Eidens D, et al. A strong candidate for the breast and ovarian cancer susceptibility gene BRCA1. Science 1994; 266:66–71.

[4] Wooster R, Bignell G, Lancaster J, et al. Identification of the breast cancer susceptibility gene BRCA2. Nature 1995;378:789–92.

[5] Szabo CI, King MC. Population genetics of BRCA1 and BRCA2. Am J Hum Genet 1997;60: 1013–20.

[6] Serova O, Mazoyer S, Puget N, et al. Mutations in BRCA1 and BRCA2 in breast cancer families: are there more breast cancer susceptibility genes? Am J Hum Genet 1997;60:486–95.

[7] Ford D, Easton DF, Bishop DT, et al. Risks of cancer in BRCA1-mutation carriers. Breast Cancer Linkage Consortium. Lancet 1994;343:692–5.

[8] Antoniou A, Pharoah PD, Narod S, et al. Average risks of breast and ovarian cancer associated with BRCA1 or BRCA2 mutations detected in case series unselected for family history: a combined analysis of 22 studies. Am J Hum Genet 2003; 72:1117–30.

[9] Armes JE, Egan AJ, Southey MC, et al. The histologic phenotypes of breast carcinoma occurring before age 40 years in women with and without BRCA1 or BRCA2 germline mutations: a population-based study. Cancer 1998;83:2335–45.

[10] Lakhani SR, Jacquemire J, Sloane JP, et al. Multifactorial analysis of differences between sporadic breast cancers and cancers involving BRCA1 and BRCA2 mutations. J Natl Cancer Inst 1998;90: 1138–45.

[11] Marcus JN, Watson P, Page DL, et al. Hereditary breast cancer: pathobiology, prognosis, and BRCA1 and BRCA2 gene linkage. Cancer 1996; 77:697–709.

[12] Breast Cancer Linkage Consortium. Pathology of familial breast cancer: differences between breast cancers in carriers of BRCA1 or BRCA2 mutations and sporadic cases. Lancet 1997;349: 1505–10.

[13] Vasen HF, Haites NE, Evans DG, et al. Current policies for surveillance and management in women at risk of breast and ovarian cancer: a survey among 16 European family cancer clinics. European Familial Breast Cancer Collaborative Group. Eur J Cancer 1998;34:1922–6.

[14] Burke W, Daly M, Garber J, et al. Recommendations for follow-up care of individuals with an inherited predisposition to cancer. II. BRCA1 and BRCA2. Cancer Genetics Studies Consortium. JAMA 1997;277:997–1003.

[15] Metcalfe K, Lynch HT, Ghadirian P, et al. Contralateral breast cancer in BRCA1 and BRCA2 mutation carriers. J Clin Oncol 2004;22:2328–35.

[16] Hoskins KF, Stopfer JE, Calzone KA, et al. Assessment and counseling for women with a family history of breast cancer. A guide for clinicians. JAMA 1995;273:577–85.

[17] Metcalfe KA, Goel V, Lickley L, et al. Prophylactic bilateral mastectomy: patterns of practice. Cancer 2002;95:236–42.

[18] Hartmann LC, Schaid DJ, Woods JE, et al. Efficacy of bilateral prophylactic mastectomy in women with a family history of breast cancer. N Engl J Med 1999;340:77–84.

[19] Meijers-Heijboer H, van Geel B, van Putten WL, et al. Breast cancer after prophylactic bilateral

mastectomy in women with a BRCA1 or BRCA2 mutation. N Engl J Med 2001;345(3):159–64.

[20] Rebbeck TR, Friebel T, Lynch HT, et al. Bilateral prophylactic mastectomy reduces breast cancer risk in BRCA1 and BRCA2 mutation carriers: the PROSE Study Group. J Clin Oncol 2004;22: 1055–62.

[21] Foulkes WD, Metcalfe K, Hanna W, et al. Disruption of the expected positive correlation between breast tumor size and lymph node status in BRCA1-related breast carcinoma. Cancer 2003; 98(8):1569–77.

[22] Kerlikowske K, Grady D, Barclay J, et al. Positive predictive value of screening mammography by age and family history of breast cancer. JAMA 1993;270:2444–50.

[23] Zhong Q, Chen CF, Chen PL, et al. BRCA1 facilitates microhomology-mediated end joining of DNA double strand breaks. J Biol Chem 2002; 277:28641–7.

[24] Somasundaram K. Breast cancer gene 1 (BRCA1): role in cell cycle regulation and DNA repair—perhaps through transcription. J Cell Biochem 2003; 88:1084–91.

[25] Sharan SK, Morimatsu M, Albrecht U, et al. Embryonic lethality and radiation hypersensitivity mediated by Rad51 in mice lacking BRCA2. Nature 1997;386:804–10.

[26] Alpert TE, Haffty BG. Conservative management of breast cancer in BRCA1/2 mutation carriers. Clin Breast Cancer 2004;5:37–42.

[27] Kirova YM, Stoppa-Lyonnet D, Savignoni A, et al, for the Institut Curie Breast Cancer Study Group. Risk of breast cancer recurrence and contralateral breast cancer in relation to BRCA1 and BRCA2 mutation status following breast-conserving surgery and radiotherapy. Eur J Cancer [Epub August 2005].

[28] Moller P, Borg A, Evans DG, et al. Survival in prospectively ascertained familial breast cancer: analysis of a series stratified by tumour characteristics, BRCA mutations and oophorectomy. Int J Cancer 2005;41(15):2304–11.

[29] Robson M, Gilewski T, Haas B, et al. BRCA-associated breast cancer in young women. J Clin Oncol 1998;16:1642–9.

[30] Robson M, Levin D, Federici M, et al. Breast conservation therapy for invasive breast cancer in Ashkenazi women with BRCA gene founder mutations. J Natl Cancer Inst 1999;91:2112–7.

[31] Veronesi A, de Giacomi C, Magri MD, et al. Familial breast cancer: characteristics and outcome of BRCA 1-2 positive and negative cases. BMC Cancer 2005;5:70.

[32] Kuhl CK, Schmutzler RK, Leutner CC, et al. Breast MR imaging screening in 192 women proved or suspected to be carriers of a breast cancer susceptibility gene: preliminary results. Radiology 2000;215:267–79.

[33] Brekelmans CT, Seynaeve C, Bartels CC, et al. Effectiveness of breast cancer surveillance in BRCA1/2 gene mutation carriers and women with high familial risk. J Clin Oncol 2001;19: 924–30.

[34] Scheuer L, Kauff ND, Robson M, et al. Outcome of preventive surgery and screening for breast and ovarian cancer in BRCA mutation carriers. J Clin Oncol 2002;20:1260–8.

[35] Gui GP, Hogben RK, Walsh G, et al. The incidence of breast cancer from screening women according to predicted family history risk: does annual clinical examination add to mammography? Eur J Cancer 2001;37:1668–73.

[36] Komenaka IK, Ditkoff BA, Joseph KA, et al. The development of interval breast malignancies in patients with BRCA mutations. Cancer 2004; 100:2079–83.

[37] Stoutjesdijk MJ, Boetes C, Jager GJ, et al. Magnetic resonance imaging and mammography in women with a hereditary risk of breast cancer. J Natl Cancer Inst 2001;93:1095–102.

[38] Warner E, Plewes DB, Shumak RS, et al. Comparison of breast magnetic resonance imaging, mammography, and ultrasound for surveillance of women at high risk for hereditary breast cancer. J Clin Oncol 2001;19:3524–31.

[39] Warner E, Plewes DB, Hill KA, et al. Surveillance of BRCA1 and BRCA2 mutation carriers with magnetic resonance imaging, ultrasound, mammography, and clinical breast examination. JAMA 2004;292:1317–25.

[40] Kriege M, Brekelmans CT, Boetes C, et al. Magnetic Resonance Imaging Screening Study Group. Efficacy of MRI and mammography for breast-cancer screening in women with a familial or genetic predisposition. N Engl J Med 2004; 351:427–37.

[41] Podo F, Sardanelli F, Canese R, et al. The Italian multi-centre project on evaluation of MRI and other imaging modalities in early detection of breast cancer in subjects at high genetic risk. J Exp Clin Cancer Res 2002;21:115–24.

[42] Robson M, Morris EA, Kauff N, et al. Breast cancer screening utilizing magnetic resonance imaging (MRI) in carriers of BRCA mutations [abstract]. Proc Am Soc Clin Oncol 2003;22:91.

[43] Trecate G, Vergnaghi D, Bergonzi S, et al. Breast MRI screening in patients with increased familial and/or genetic risk for breast cancer: a preliminary experience. Tumori 2003;89:125–31.

[44] Tilanus-Linthorst M, Verhoog L, Obdeijn IM, et al. A BRCA1/2 mutation, high breast density and prominent pushing margins of a tumor independently contribute to a frequent false-negative mammography. Int J Cancer 2002; 102:91–5.

[45] Kuhl CK, Schrading S, Leutner CK, et al. Mammography, breast ultrasound, and magnetic resonance imaging for surveillance of women at high genetic risk for breast cancer. J Clin Oncol 2005;23:8469–76.

[46] Kuhl CK, Schrading S, Weigel S, et al. Die "EVA-Studie": Evaluierung der Leistungsfähigkeit diagnostischer Verfahren (Mammographie,

Sonographie, MRT) zur sekundären und tertiären Prävention des familiären Mammakarzinoms—Zwischenergebnisse nach der ersten Hälfte der Förderungsperiode. Fortschr Röntgenstr 2005;177:818–27.

[47] Leach MO, Boggis CR, Dixon AK, et al. Screening with magnetic resonance imaging and mammography of a UK population at high familial risk of breast cancer: a prospective multicentre cohort study (MARIBS). Lancet 2005;365:1769–78.

[48] Kuhl CK, Schrading S, Leutner CC, et al. Surveillance of "high risk" women with proven or suspected familial (hereditary) breast cancer: first mid-term results of a multi-modality clinical screening trial [abstract]. Proc Am Soc Clin Oncol 2003;22:2.

MAGNETIC
RESONANCE
IMAGING CLINICS

Magn Reson Imaging Clin N Am 14 (2006) 403–409

ELSEVIER
SAUNDERS

Do We Need Randomized Controlled Clinical Trials to Evaluate the Clinical Impact of Breast MR Imaging?

Bruce J. Hillman, MD[a,b,c,*]

- Imaging and cancer—the potential applications of breast MR imaging
- The clinical research hierarchy and the assessment of breast MR imaging
- The special case of screening
- Modeling and decision analysis
- Summary
- References

Worldwide, mammography is the standard technology used in the screening and diagnosis of breast cancer. It has been well shown in numerous large, population-based studies to be an effective means of detecting breast cancer at an earlier stage than physical examination. The use of mammography reduces the mortality rate from breast cancer [1–5].

Increasingly, mammographic detection and diagnosis is being supplemented—and in some settings even supplanted—by MR imaging of the breast. Single institutional studies and early multicenter clinical trials are finding that breast MR imaging detects more breast cancers than mammography [6–18]. In many ways, MR imaging is also a more versatile technology. As will be detailed below, breast MR imaging can be used not only for early detection and diagnosis, but for the complete gamut of potential applications of imaging to the care of breast cancer.

While preliminary reports of the successful use of breast MR imaging are encouraging, it must be remembered that this is almost always the case with the assessment of new imaging technologies by researchers who are expert in its use and whose careers are tied to the technology. Subsequently, more rigorous research, including the evaluation of how a technology performs in more general practice often is disappointing in comparison. Breast MR imaging has yet to undergo this level of scrutiny, although larger trials of various applications are now underway. These trials—and subsequent ones—must necessarily go beyond measuring such metrics as sensitivity, specificity, and the area under the receiver operating characteristic curve to determining the impact breast MR imaging has on clinical care. Ultimately, breast MR imaging will have to show, in rigorously designed, generalizable clinical trials, that it significantly reduces patient morbidity and mortality from breast cancer if it is to earn a permanent place in the imaging armamentarium for this disease.

This article provides examples of how this could be done by describing trials reflecting the thinking

Dr. Hillman is the Principal Investigator of a grant from the National Cancer Institute that funds the American College of Radiology Imaging Network (ACRIN).

a Department of Radiology, University of Virginia, PO Box 800170, Charlottesville, VA 22908, USA
b Department of Public Health Services, University of Virginia, PO Box 800170, Charlottesville, VA 22908, USA
c American College of Radiology Imaging Network, Philadelphia, PA, USA
* Radiology-UVAHS, PO Box 800170, Charlottesville VA 22908.
E-mail address: bjh8a@virginia.edu

doi:10.1016/j.mric.2006.07.008

of researchers working with the American College of Radiology Imaging Network (ACRIN), a National Cancer Institute (NCI)–funded cooperative group engaged in multicenter clinical trials of imaging as it relates to cancer, including breast cancer.

Imaging and cancer—the potential applications of breast MR imaging

Broadly speaking, there are four principal applications of medical imaging to the care of cancer:

- **Screening, also known as early detection**
- **Diagnosis and staging**
- **Image-guided treatment**
- **Follow-up of treatment to determine if the treatment was successful**

Potentially, breast MR imaging could be applicable to all four of these applications. The design of a clinical study and its endpoints will vary according to which of these applications is being addressed, as well as with the goals of the research.

With respect to screening, there has been some research into breast MR imaging screening of specialized populations [19–22]—those known to be more prone to the development of breast cancer, such as individuals with the *BRCA* genes or women who previously have had breast cancer. A major multicenter trial of this application by ACRIN that focuses on the number of cancers identified closed accrual in 2004. Subjects are now in the follow-up phase (Constance Lehman, MD, University of Washington, personal communication). The principle objections to the expanded use of MR imaging screening for breast cancer are its high cost and that it has not been definitively shown to reduce breast cancer–specific mortality—the sine qua non for screening tests. This topic is discussed in much more detail later in this article.

Breast MR imaging also could be used to determine whether a mass identified on mammography or ultrasonography actually represents a cancer. Dynamic contrast-enhanced (DCE)–MR imaging techniques have been established to address this application [10]. Whole-body MR imaging might serve as a "one-stop shop" to determine whether there are local or distant metastases. Such staging is necessary to determine which therapy is appropriate for any given case.

Several companies and academic institutions are developing technologies that would use MR imaging to guide treatment for breast cancer (Mitchell Schnall, MD, PhD, University of Pennsylvania, personal communication, 2006). MR imaging has the potential to exquisitely differentiate cancer from surrounding tissue and to determine to what extent treatment is affecting cancerous versus normal tissues. ACRIN is in the concept development phase of assessing such a technology that uses focused ultrasound scan to extracutaneously ablate breast cancers. This article does not consider any further treatment trials, because they are quite different from trials of diagnostic technologies and outside the scope of this forum.

MR imaging already is proving useful in determining whether treatment for breast cancer has been effective. Traditionally, this has meant sequential anatomic measurement of primary tumors or metastases on scans performed at distant intervals. However, there is general dissatisfaction with this technique from all sides. Performing the measurements is tedious. The measurements tend to be poorly reproducible.

There are little data to support that linear or even volume measurements correlate well with patient outcomes. Much better would be a physiologic or metabolic test that would determine the impact of treatment on the disease and serve as a timely, reliable intermediate marker (sometimes called a biomarker) of the effectiveness of therapy. Such a test using MR imaging to evaluate treatment for advanced breast cancer is being assessed as part of a collaborative trial involving ACRIN and one of the National Cancer Institute's (NCI's) therapeutic cooperative groups, the Cancer and Leukemia Group B (CALGB; Nola Hyton, PhD, University of California San Francisco, personal communication, 2005). This trial uses three to four sequential DCE–MR imaging—a test that evaluates a breast cancer's circulation—during a course of neoadjuvant therapy, paired with simultaneous core biopsy, to determine whether the DCE–MR imaging result correlates with tissue changes and eventual patient outcome.

The clinical research hierarchy and the assessment of breast MR imaging

Determining how to evaluate breast MR imaging—that is, what research design to use and what endpoints to focus on—is a complex endeavor. To complicate matters, breast MR imaging is a rapidly evolving technology that is just now disseminating widely into clinical practice in all its potential applications. This too has an effect on what is feasible and practical in the way of research. Different research designs require vastly different investments and take varying amounts of time from conception to completion. It makes little sense to consider a cost-effectiveness analysis of a technology that is in rapid flux, whereas this may be exactly the correct approach for a mature technology in which the reader performance (ie, accuracy) is well established. This is an important consideration to ensure that whatever research design is chosen, the result will be germane to clinical practice when it finally emerges.

To address the question of what research designs to use for which breast MR imaging questions, it is useful to return to the basics—the hierarchy of clinical research in diagnostic imaging [23,24]. When imaging technologies are first introduced, there is usually a period in which the technology is seeking applications in clinical practice. The imaging literature reflects this, as there is usually a flurry of articles detailing case reports and case series in which the technology has been used. The biases of such publications— particularly selection, validation, and investigator biases—have been well detailed in the literature [25,26].

Scientific clinical research begins with evaluating "diagnostic efficacy." This level of research asks the question, "How well do interpreters of images derived from the technology distinguish between normal and abnormal cases?" Measurements for this level of the hierarchy include ones with which all radiologists should be familiar—sensitivity, specificity, positive and negative predictive values, and receiver operating characteristic curve (ROC) analysis. As noted above, there have been a number of studies already that have shown encouraging results for breast MR imaging with regard to diagnostic efficacy. Generally, such studies use a paired design, wherein each subject receives both breast MR imaging and a comparison imaging technology (most often mammography). This is a more efficient approach than using randomization, because each subject can serve as his or her own control, allowing for smaller sample sizes and more rapid conduct of the trial.

Although clearly a diagnostic test must have superior characteristics of observer performance, this does not guarantee that using the technology will have a positive impact on patient care. To evaluate whether breast MR imaging affects the care a patient receives, we must ascend to the next two levels of the clinical research hierarchy, "diagnostic thinking efficacy" and "therapeutic thinking efficacy." The former refers to how performing a test affects the referring physician's diagnostic considerations, whereas the latter refers to what treatment he or she is contemplating. Research investigating these considerations is relatively scant for medical imaging in general and has not been a significant focus of research on breast MR imaging to date. Research at this level generally uses a pre- versus posttesting design [27,28] in which referring clinicians are asked to express their diagnostic or therapeutic considerations before and after the performance of the diagnostic test. The investigators measure the change that occurs in diagnostic or therapeutic thinking.

Obviously, all of this is important, but what society really wants to know is the extent to which the use of an imaging technology positively changes health and what expenditures will it consume in doing so. This genre of research goes by the buzz word, *outcomes research*. Outcomes research studies are quite rare in medical imaging because of the nature of medical imaging and because of the incentives and reward structure for doing medical imaging research. With regard to the former, imaging is, for most medical scenarios, but a single step in a chain of diagnostic and therapeutic interventions that ultimately lead to a health outcome. It can be very difficult to separate out the specific effect of the imaging test on that outcome from the effects of all of the other diagnostic and therapeutic interventions. The fact that doing this kind of research is complex, necessarily multidisciplinary, time-consuming, and expensive—and that there are significant risks that the research will lead to naught—goes counter to the imaging research culture. A cursory evaluation of the radiology literature shows that the majority of what constitutes radiology research is single institutional research by groups of radiologists using internal funding in their spare time. The tangible incentives to do imaging research support this phenomenon. Few radiologists invest in the years of research training necessary to learn to lead multidisciplinary research teams, and the reward system of promotion and tenure, travel, and lionization seems to favor high quantity over quality.

The critical health outcome of interest with respect to breast MR imaging is breast cancer–specific mortality. As a generalization, if we are interested in knowing the impact of breast MR imaging relative to current practice on mortality, it is necessary to adopt the randomized, controlled clinical trial (RCT) approach. This is because if all subjects receive both technologies, it is not possible to distinguish whether an observed positive effect is attributable to one technology or the other. The same is generally true of investigating cost, although a novel design being used in the ACRIN Digital Mammographic Imaging Screening Trial (DMIST) shows that if our goals in this regard are limited, this assertion is not an absolute (Etta Pisano, MD, University of North Carolina, personal communication, 2005).

The special case of screening

Breast MR imaging has been proposed as a screening technology, either for the general population or for special populations that are at elevated risk for contracting breast cancer. The word "screening," in this context implies the routine, systematic, sequential breast MR imaging of asymptomatic individuals, the goal of which is to detect breast cancer in an early, preclinical phase. For screening to be successful, this early-phase detection must portend a better outcome than if diagnosis occurs later in the course of disease. In addition, the positive effect must occur at a cost that society can afford. Opinions about what society can afford differ, but the price is set generally at around $50,000 per quality-adjusted year-of-life saved (QALYS).

One might imagine a number of potential endpoints for screening studies. Early studies often focus on the numbers of additional cancers detected beyond what is found with the standard, or conventional, technology. Another endpoint that frequently attracts interest is "stage shift"—the finding that a greater preponderance of cancers identified by screening are found at lower, potentially more curable stages. Screening advocates point to quality-of-life measures, such as relief of anxiety, and there are standardized, validated methods for measuring these types of endpoints. All of these endpoints can be measured by a variety of observational approaches that do not necessarily require randomization, although rigorous investigators must account for potential biases in their observational designs.

However, although these endpoints are interesting, there is general agreement that if we are considering instituting a population-based breast MR imaging screening program, which inevitably is very expensive even when dealing with less-expensive technologies than breast MR imaging, the principal benefit needs to be a reduction in the mortality rate relative to our current screening regimen based on mammography (ie, incremental benefit). This benefit cannot be inferred from other endpoints, such as those listed above, because of specific biases that are associated with observational studies of screening, notably, lead-time bias, length bias, and overdiagnosis [29,30].

Lead-time bias refers to the possibility that diagnosing a cancer in the preclinical phase may lead to longer survival simply because we learn about the disease earlier, but, in fact, death occurs at exactly the same point as if we diagnosed the condition once signs and symptoms occur. The patient appears to live longer, but, in fact, this is a mirage. Hence, "breast cancer survival" (ie, average length of time until death after diagnosis) is an inaccurate proxy for what we really wish to know—does breast MR imaging screening reduce the "breast cancer–specific mortality rate" (ie, number of deaths per thousand population per annum).

Breast cancer is a heterogeneous disease, with high variability in aggressiveness—from very indolent tumors that will not affect patients in their lifetimes to rapidly progressive tumors that metastasize early and lead to rapid death. This biological concept is fundamental to understanding length bias and overdiagnosis. With regard to length bias, screening naturally selects for the more frequent detection of indolent tumors than aggressive ones because indolent tumors have a longer preclinical phase, during which they are subject to detection by screening. As a result, on average, patients whose breast cancer is detected by screening are more likely to have an extended course (ie, longer survival) than those whose disease is symptomatic at the time of diagnosis.

Finally, overdiagnosis refers to the detection of breast cancer that will not affect the subject during their lifetime. There are two possibilities in this regard: either the cancer is static or extremely slow growing, or death by some other cause intervenes before the time at which the breast cancer would kill the patient. In a sense, overdiagnosis could be considered an extreme case of length bias.

The astute reader will note that all three major screening biases described above act to skew results from observational trials in the same direction. They all make screening appear to be more effective than it really is. Thus, if we really are to learn whether breast MR imaging reduces the mortality rate to a greater extent than mammography, a research design must be identified that obviates these and other potential biases; this would be the RCT [31].

The RCT is the gold standard for research on therapeutic innovations but, for reasons detailed above, has been used little in medical imaging. Still, for the purposes of a comprehensive evaluation of a proposed screening modality's impact on disease-specific mortality and cost, performing an RCT is ultimately a necessity. An RCT allows that there are not only known biases, such as those described above, but potentially unknown biases that could skew the results of observational research and lead us astray with regard to practice recommendations (the principal goal of doing clinical research). An RCT helps avoid this pitfall through the process of assigning subjects randomly to one or another (but not both) competing technologies. In essence, an RCT acknowledges biases may exist but allows that they will be ameliorated by their effects being equally distributed between the arms of the trial.

Although the verity of conducting an RCT for breast MR imaging is incontrovertible, there are significant problems with this approach. RCTs are difficult to design, ponderous, and time consuming. Because even in a high-risk population, such as screening only patients with previous breast cancer or positive BRCA testing, the disease is rare in contrast to the majority of subjects who will be normal; thus, large samples are required to attain a meaningful result. Such large studies tend to be very expensive and time-consuming; subjects need to be screened repeatedly and followed over an extended period to allow for the interval development of cancers. Finally, there are important ethical considerations. Simplistically, the two (or more) arms of the trial must be in "equipoise," which means that the current state of research, as reviewed by unbiased observers (ie, not investigators attached to one or the other technology), supports the equivalence of the two arms (prospectively, in this case, breast MR imaging and mammography).

Illustrative of these points is ACRIN's National Lung Screening Trial (NLST), an RCT that compares chest x-ray and chest CT as screening approaches to decrease lung cancer–specific mortality. Some observational studies suggest that CT screening confers an incremental benefit in survival (remember, this is not the same as the mortality rate) [32,33], although there is conflicting evidence on whether it truly confers a stage shift to support this conclusion [34]. It is unclear whether the observational studies of screening CT reflect a real benefit or the biases associated with nonexperimental studies of screening. In addition, there is a high false-positive rate, so there is real concern about the frequency of unnecessary workups and inappropriate treatment that CT screening might engender, including concerns about associated high costs. Recognizing the potential health and financial consequences of unproven but disseminated CT screening for lung cancer, the NCI funded the NLST, an RCT that is designed to determine whether chest x-ray or CT screening for lung cancer is cost-effective for high risk individuals (ie, those who are older than 55 years and have an extensive smoking history). The trial requires a sample of 50,000 high-risk subjects assigned randomly to screening by one or the other technology for 3 consecutive years, and followed up for 2 additional years, to answer the question, at an 80% level of certainty: "Does one or the other screening technology reduce lung cancer mortality by at least 20%." The trial also assesses the screening and downstream costs, the impact of screening on quality of life and smoking habits, and a number of other screening-related issues. Biospecimens are being collected annually on a subsample of 10,000 subjects for future research on genetic predictors of lung cancer. With the design and ramp-up phases, recruitment of the 30 participating sites, the handling of regulatory issues, and the time needed to analyze such complex data, the trial will take at least 8 years to conduct and cost approximately $200 million.

Consider the analogies. A screening trial of breast MR imaging—even one focused on a selected high-risk population—might well need to be as large and as expensive as the NLST, and might take as long to conduct. A screening study of the general population would be far more expensive, requiring a greater number of subjects, because of the lower incidence of disease among normal-risk individuals. But, as noted above, in the absence of such a trial, the positive biases associated with the types of observational research being conducted today might well lead us astray into incorrectly believing that breast MR imaging is beneficial, when in fact a substantial benefit in reduced mortality does not exist.

Modeling and decision analysis

Given the time and money involved, it should be considered whether conducting an RCT would be worthwhile. Fortunately, there are formalized methods that use "virtual" patient cohorts, generically referred to as *decision analysis* [35,36]. Decision analysis requires the development of a clinical model that generically reflects the pathway through which women would progress depending on characteristics intrinsic to the women themselves, the incidence and biological nature of breast cancer, the diagnostic test or tests to which virtual women are assigned, the observer performance of those tests, possible treatments, the possible outcomes, and the utilities (ie, relative personal values) subjects would assign to those outcomes. In essence, the model is a simplification of real life and as a result cannot necessarily be considered a true reflection of how competing tests might perform in an RCT. Despite this, decision analysis can give us significant insight into whether a prospective new technology is at least in the competitive range of providing an incremental benefit at an acceptable cost. In addition, the method can point out areas of uncertainty that can instruct the design of a trial and help focus a trial so that it is less complex and hence less expensive.

Summary

To address the title of this article directly, "Do we need RCTs to assess the clinical impact of breast MR imaging?" It depends. This is not a very satisfying answer, but it is the only one possible. The appropriate design for research on the clinical value of breast MR imaging depends on the application being studied and the endpoint(s) of interest. What is most desirable in the way of research must be balanced against its practicality.

References

[1] Leung JW. Screening mammography reduces morbidity of breast cancer treatment. AJR Am J Roentgenol 2005;184:1508–9.

[2] Otto SJ, Fracheboud J, Looman CW, et al. National Evaluation Team for Breast Cancer Screening. Initiation of population-based mammography screening in Dutch municipalities and effect on breast-cancer mortality: a systematic review. Lancet 2003;361:1411–7.

[3] Tabar L, Yen MF, Vitak B, et al. Mammography screening and mortality in breast cancer patients: 20-year follow-up before and after introduction of screening. Lancet 2003;361:1405–10.

[4] Nystrom L, Andersson I, Bjurstam N, et al. Long-term effects of mammography screening: updated overview of the Swedish randomised trials. Lancet 2002;359:909–19.

[5] Kopans DB. The most recent breast cancer screening controversy about whether mammographic screening benefits women at any age: nonsense and nonscience. AJR Am J Roentgenol 2003;180:21–6.

[6] Morris EA, Liberman L, Ballon DJ, et al. MRI of occult breast carcinoma in a high-risk population. AJR Am J Roentgenol 2003;181:619–26.

[7] Liberman L, Morris EA, Dershaw DD, et al. MR imaging of the ipsilateral breast in women with percutaneously proven breast cancer. AJR Am J Roentgenol 2003;180:901–10.

[8] Liberman L, Morris EA, Kim CM, et al. MR imaging findings in the contralateral breast of women with recently diagnosed breast cancer. AJR Am J Roentgenol 2003;180:333–41.

[9] Fischer U, Zachariae O, Baum F, et al. The influence of preoperative MRI of the breasts on recurrence rate in patients with breast cancer. Eur Radiol 2004;14:1725–31.

[10] Bluemke DA, Gatsonis CA, Chen MH, et al. Magnetic resonance imaging of the breast prior to biopsy. JAMA 2004;292:2735–42.

[11] Lee JM, Orel SG, Czerniecki BJ, et al. MRI before reexcision surgery in patients with breast cancer. AJR Am J Roentgenol 2004;182:473–80.

[12] Lehman CD, Blume JD, Weatherall P, et al. Screening women at high risk for breast cancer with mammography and magnetic resonance imaging. Cancer 2005;103:1898–905.

[13] Hylton N. Magnetic resonance imaging of the breast: opportunities to improve breast cancer management. J Clin Oncol 2005;23:1678–84.

[14] Hwang ES, Kinkel K, Esserman LJ, et al. Magnetic resonance imaging in patients diagnosed with ductal carcinoma-in-situ: value in the diagnosis of residual disease, occult invasion, and multicentricity. Ann Surg Oncol 2003;10:381–8.

[15] Wallace AM, Daniel BL, Jeffrey SS, et al. Rates of reexcision for breast cancer after magnetic resonance imaging-guided bracket wire localization. J Am Coll Surg 2005;200:527–37.

[16] Meisamy S, Bolan PJ, Baker EH, et al. Neoadjuvant chemotherapy of locally advanced breast cancer: predicting response with in vivo (1)H MR spectroscopy–a pilot study at 4 T. Radiology 2004;233:424–31.

[17] Londero V, Bazzocchi M, Del Frate C, et al. Locally advanced breast cancer: comparison of mammography, sonography and MR imaging in evaluation of residual disease in women receiving neoadjuvant chemotherapy. Eur Radiol 2004;14:1371–9.

[18] Partridge SC, Gibbs JE, Lu Y, et al. Accuracy of MR imaging for revealing residual breast cancer in patients who have undergone neoadjuvant chemotherapy. AJR Am J Roentgenol 2002;179:1193–9.

[19] Kuhl CK, Schmutzler RK, Leutner CC, et al. Breast MR imaging screening in 192 women proved or suspected to be carriers of a breast cancer susceptibility gene: preliminary results. Radiology 2000;215:267–79.

[20] Stoutjesdijk MJ, Boetes C, Jager GJ, et al. Magnetic resonance imaging and mammography in women with a hereditary risk of breast cancer. J Natl Cancer Inst 2001;93:1095–102.

[21] Warner E, Plewes DB, Hill KA, et al. Surveillance of BRCA1 and BRCA2 mutation carriers with magnetic resonance imaging, ultrasound, mammography, and clinical breast examination. JAMA 2004;292:1317.

[22] Kriege M, Brekelmans CT, Boetes C, et al. Magnetic Resonance Imaging Screening Study Group. Efficacy of MRI and mammography for breast-cancer screening in women with a familial or genetic predisposition. N Engl J Med 2004; 351:427–37.

[23] Fryback DG, Thornbury R. The Efficacy of diagnostic imaging. Med Decis Making 1991;11:88–94.

[24] Hillman BJ. Outcomes research and cost-effectiveness analysis for diagnostic imaging. Radiology 1994;193:307–10.

[25] Hillman BJ. Critical thinking: deciding whether to incorporate into practice the recommendations of radiology publications and presentations. Am J Roentagenol 2000;174:943–6.

[26] Black WC. How to evaluate the radiology literature. AJR Am J Roentgenol 1990;154:17–22.

[27] Thornbury JR, Fryback DG, Edwards W. Likelihood ratios as a measure of diagnostic usefulness of excretory urogram information. Radiology 1975;114:561–5.

[28] Omary RA, Kaplan PA, Dussault RG, et al. The impact of ankle radiography on the diagnosis and management of acute ankle injuries. Acad Radiol 1996;3:758–65.

[29] Black WC. Overdiagnosis: an underrecognized cause of confusion and harm in cancer screening. J Natl Cancer Inst 2000;92:1280–2.

[30] Black WC, Ling A. Is earlier diagnosis really better? The misleading effects of lead time and length biases. AJR Am J Roentgenol 1990;155:625–30.

[31] Kopans DB, Monsees B, Feig SA. Screening for cancer: when is it valid? – Lessons from the mammography experience. Radiology 2003;229:319–27.

[32] Henschke CI, McCauley DI, Yankelevitz DF, et al. Early Lung Cancer Action Project: overall design and findings from baseline screening. Lancet 1999;354:99–105.

[33] Sone S, Takashima S, Li F, et al. Mass screening for lung cancer with mobile spiral computed tomography scanner. Lancet 1998;351:1242–5.

[34] Swensen SJ, Jett JR, Hartman TE, et al. CT screening for lung cancer: five-year prospective experience. Radiology 2005;235:259–65.

[35] Mahadevia PJ, Fleisher LA, Frick KD, et al. Lung cancer screening with helical CT in older adult smokers. JAMA 2003;289:313–22.

[36] Beinfeld MT, Wittenberg E, Gazelle GS. Cost-effectiveness of whole body CT screening. Radiology 2005;234:415–22.

ELSEVIER
SAUNDERS

MAGNETIC
RESONANCE
IMAGING CLINICS

Magn Reson Imaging Clin N Am 14 (2006) 411–425

MRI-Guided Percutaneous Biopsy of Breast Lesions: Materials, Techniques, Success Rates, and Management in Patients with Suspected Radiologic-Pathologic Mismatch

Daniel Floery, MD, Thomas H. Helbich, MD*

In the last decade, contrast-enhanced MR imaging of the breast has gained recognition as a valuable adjunct to mammography and ultrasound in the detection of breast carcinomas. There is general agreement among investigators that the sensitivity of breast MR imaging is excellent, ranging between 88% and 100%. MR imaging enables the identification of otherwise clinically, sonographically, and mammographically occult lesions and allows a precise determination of the extent of the disease, including the presence of multifocal or multicentric disease [1–7]. Rapid enhancement and early wash-out are generally observed in breast carcinomas, but there are exceptions to this pattern. Certain carcinomas, particularly lobular cancer and carcinoma in situ, may enhance slowly or not at all. On the other hand, some enhancement may be observed in benign lesions such as fibroadenomas. The specificity of MR imaging of the breast has been variable, ranging from 37% to 97% [1,4,5,7,8]. Despite the use of

Department of Radiology, Medical University of Vienna–AKH WIEN, Waehringer Guertel 18-20, 1090 Vienna, Austria
* Corresponding author.
E-mail address: thomas.helbich@akhwien.at (T.H. Helbich).

1064-9689/06/$ – see front matter © 2006 Elsevier Inc. All rights reserved. doi:10.1016/j.mric.2006.10.002
mri.theclinics.com

several criteria in the classification of MR imaging–detected lesions (MR imaging lexicon [9,10]) and the interpretation of contrast-enhancement kinetics (ROI [11–13]), suspicious BIRADS IV and V lesions still require histologic diagnosis.

Two different approaches to the histologic verification of MR imaging–detected breast lesions are feasible. The first is MR imaging–guided needle-localized open breast biopsy [14–17]. Although open breast biopsy yields good results, the surgery is costly, invasive, and associated with a certain perioperative risk. As an alternative, percutaneous breast biopsy techniques under MR imaging guidance have been developed. Under mammographic and sonographic guidance, percutaneous biopsy techniques have already been carefully evaluated and have been shown to be safe and accurate methods [18–22]. When compared with open breast biopsy, percutaneous biopsy is less invasive, faster, and can be performed at lower costs [20].

This review focuses on the currently available devices and techniques for MR imaging–guided percutaneous breast biopsy and reports their achievable diagnostic accuracy. Technical success rates and strategies for patient management after the interventional procedure are outlined. The discussion also includes new developments in MR imaging–guided minimally invasive therapeutic interventions, as well as the potential for research opportunities and directions.

Patient selection and interventional planning

For MR imaging–guided percutaneous breast biopsy, accurate pre-interventional planning and careful patient selection are highly recommended to guarantee a successful procedure. In particular, this process includes strict criteria for the indications and analysis of diagnostic MR imaging of the breast.

Indications for MR imaging–guided breast biopsy

If a diagnostic MR imaging study of the breast identifies a suspicious lesion, every effort should be made to re-identify the lesion on conventional modalities such as mammography or ultrasound [23]. If the lesion can be clearly identified on mammography or ultrasound, biopsy should be performed using one of these guiding modalities; however, second-look ultrasound fails to identify a sonographic correlate in as many as 77% of MR imaging–detected lesions referred for biopsy [24,25].

Percutaneous biopsy is most often used for the evaluation of BIRADS IV lesions, for which a malignant rate of 30% to 50% is reported in studies with mammographically or sonographically guided biopsy [18]. In BIRADS V lesions, needle biopsy has revealed a malignant rate of almost 90%; therefore, the use of needle biopsy depends on the clinical setting. Percutaneous needle biopsy in BIRADS V lesions is indicated in instances of planned preoperative chemotherapy and as an alternative to diagnostic surgical biopsy when a second surgical procedure is planned. For a one-stage therapeutic strategy, including the diagnosis of carcinoma with a frozen section, percutaneous biopsy is not indicated in BIRADS V lesions.

For BIRADS III (probably benign) lesions, 6-month short-term follow-up is recommended, because the frequency of carcinoma in these lesions is low, ranging from 0.5% to 2% [26–29]. There are a few indications for which biopsy of BIRADS III lesions may be considered, such as when follow-up is compromised or not available, in the instance of planned pregnancy, or for patient anxiety [18,20,27,30].

Patient information and consent

Before beginning the biopsy, several important points of the procedure should be explained to the patient, and written informed consent should be obtained. In addition, the patient should be informed about possible complications, such as hematomas or infections. Usually, patients tolerate the biopsy procedure well, and any discomfort is easily controlled with local anesthesia which should be performed routinely. If necessary, sedation of the patient can be performed with midazolam hydrochloride administered intravenously.

MR imaging units and pulse sequences

Magnets

Most MR-guided interventions are performed in closed MR imaging units with field strengths of 1.0 or 1.5 T. In closed magnets, only the identification of the lesion and the verification of correct needle position are performed under MR guidance. All other steps of the procedure (placement of the coaxial needle, retrieval of biopsy specimens) are performed outside the magnet (Fig. 1) [16,31–38].

Some groups have reported on MR-guided biopsies in open magnets, which are available from several manufacturers [39–44]. These units have low magnetic field strengths (0.2 to 0.5 T) and provide direct vertical or horizontal access to the patient. Open systems appear to have advantages over closed systems in that they provide direct access to the breast during the entire intervention and allow real-time monitoring of the needle insertion and placement. In addition, they allow performing interventions in the direction of the magnetic field, which minimizes susceptibility artifacts. Their low

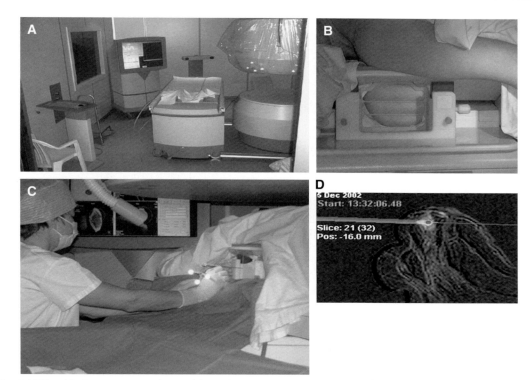

Fig. 1. MRI-guided percutaneous breast biopsy in an open magnet using a "free-hand" technique. (*A*) Interventional MR imaging suite with a magnet at the right, the mobile imaging monitor screen in the left corner of the room and the image acquisition console in the left first plan. The "optical eye" (located behind the examination table in the center) is used to record the position of the fiducials attached to the needle, providing imaging of the needle in near-real time (see *Fig. 8C*). (*B*) Patient positioning for diagnostic MRI followed by a MRI guided biopsy. The patient is in a prone position with the breast moderately compressed by a compression plate in a dedicated open breast coil. (*C*) Three stereotactic fiducials are attached to the needle. The "optical eye" records these fiducials to calculate the position of the needle. During needle positioning in the magnet room, the radiologist follows image acquisition at the monitor. (*D*) Axial T1-weighted fast gradient echo images after needle introduction and before shooting. The red line corresponds to the projected gun advancement. The green line represents the virtual needle that is displayed at the screen. The posterior part of the hyperintense lesion is marked with a red point as the target. (Courtesy of Karen Kinkel, MD, Geneva, Switzerland).

field strengths make open magnets unsuitable for diagnostic imaging, and they are not as prevalent as closed magnets. Table 1 provides a comparison of biopsy results obtained in open and closed systems.

Pulse sequences

For lesion identification, which is necessary to plan the MR-guided procedure, contrast-enhanced studies (0.1 mmol Gd-DTPA/kg) are routinely performed. The authors and others recommend using the same sequence as for the diagnostic MR imaging study. These sequences are usually two- or three-dimensional gradient-echo with and without image subtraction or with fat saturation. To save time, the number of dynamic scans can be reduced to one pre- and one or two postcontrast scans. Due to the cyclic variations of contrast enhancement, MR imaging of the breast should be performed in

the second week of the menstrual cycle. If the patient and the surgeon can accept a certain delay in the diagnostic procedure, the biopsy procedure should be planned in this time interval as well to prevent nonspecific contrast enhancement [45,46]. For rapid orientation of the needle position during the intervention, sequences should be used that allow visualization of the needle with little or no artifacts. The authors recommend using a two-dimensional gradient-echo sequence with a reduced number of slices and image matrix and a temporal resolution of less than 30 seconds [4,47,48].

Devices

Most MR imaging–guided biopsy procedures are performed with stereotactic devices that at least partially immobilize the breast during the intervention by using a compression mechanism (Fig. 2),

Table 1: **MR imaging–guided percutaneous breast biopsy: a review of the literature**

Study	Total	Technical success	MR imaging unit	Technique	Mean size	Benign	High risk	Malignant	Missed carcinomas	Underestimated carcinomas
LCBB										
Chen et al, 2004 [51]	35	34	1.5 T, C	LCBB, 14 G	Range, 3–17 mm	21	5	8	0	2
Lehman et al, 2003 [59]	5	5	1.5 T, C	LCBB, 14 G	9.5 mm	2	1	2	0	0
Kuhl et al, 2001 [35]a	59	58	1.5 T, C	LCBB, 14 G	14.6 mm	36	NG	22	1	0
Fischer et al, 1998 [36]	5	4	1.5 T,C	LCBB	Carcinomas <20 mm	3	NG	1	0	0
Kuhl et al, 1997 [34]	5	4	1.5 T,C	LCBB, 16 G	NG	0	0	4	0	0
Fischer et al, 1997 [60]	5	5	NG, C	LCBB	NG	4	0	1	NG	NG
Schneider et al, 2002 [39]	21	20	0.5 T, O	LCBB, 16 G	9.9 mm	11	1	8	0	0
Daniel et al, 2001 [43]	27	27	0.5 T, O	LCBB, 14 G	18 mm	NG	NG	NG	1	1
Sittek et al, 2000 [41]	5	5	0.2 T, O	LCBB, 16 G	NG	4	0	1	1	NG
Pfleiderer et al, 2003 [62]	14	14	1.5 T, C	LCBB, 14 G	18.6 mm	9	NG	5	1	1
VABB										
Orel, 2006 [72]	85	85	1.5 T,C	VABB, 9 G	NG	15	18	52	0 (6)	2
Liberman, 2005 [68]	98	95	1.5 T, C	VABB, 9 G	10 mm	52b	10	24	4c	3
Lehman et al, 2005 [67]	38	38	1.5 T, C	VABB, 9 G	Masses 9.3 mm	22	2	14	1	2
Liberman et al, 2003 [66]	28	27	1.5 T, C	VABB, 9 G	10 mm	20	1	6	1	1
Perlet et al, 2002 [65]	341	334	1.0/1.5 T, C	VABB, 11 G	Carcinomas 14 mm	233	17	84	0d	3
Perlet et al, 2002 [64]	206	202	1.0/1.5 T, C	VABB, 11 G	NG	144	7	51	0e	1
Heywang-Kobrunner et al, 1999 [32]	55	54	1.0 T, C	VABB, 11 G	8.4 mm	40	NG	14	0	0
FNAB										
Fischer et al, 1998 [36]	31	28	1.5 T,C	FNAB, 19.5 G	Carcinomas <20 mm	21	NG	7	0	0
Wald et al, [56]	18	11	NG	FNAB, 22 G	18 mm	11	NG	2	NG	NG

Abbreviations: C, closed magnet; FNAB, fine-needle aspiration biopsy; G, gauge; LCBB, large-core breast biopsy; NG, not given; O, open magnet; VABB, vacuum-assisted breast biopsy.
a Only cases with validation are reported.
b Further nine lesions were discordant.
c All four missed carcinomas were found among the discordant lesions.
d Seven lesions were initially missed at biopsy but were immediately recognized after the procedure.
e Four lesions were initially missed at biopsy but were immediately recognized after the procedure.

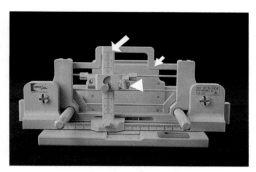

Fig. 2. Breast biopsy and compression device (Noras, Würzburg, Germany). The procedure is performed in the prone position. The breast is compressed by two compression frames with elastic bands (*small arrow*). A guiding block with a needle carrier mounted on a guiding stick allows various needle angulations and access to all parts of the breast (*large arrow*). A fluid-filled marker (*arrowhead*), which can be imaged, is used to calculate the coordinates of the lesion.

permitting precise needle placement, which is a critical factor for successful tissue sampling. There is good evidence in the literature that a high diagnostic accuracy can be achieved with stereotactic systems (Table 1). MR imaging–guided biopsies with a free-hand technique performed in closed magnets cannot be recommended. Due to insufficient fixation of the breast during the intervention, accurate sampling cannot be guaranteed.

Stereotactic systems usually consist of three main components: a compression mechanism, an imaging coil, and an aiming device. Various systems have been described in the literature that differ primarily in patient position during the intervention (supine, prone, or prone decubitus position) and the compression device (perforated plates, compression with flexible ribs) [16,33,34]. Only moderate compression of the breast is recommended, because strong compression may impair lesion enhancement and distort the anatomic structures of the breast [49]. Most stereotactic devices are designed to support biopsy equipment for large-core breast biopsy (LCBB) and vacuum-assisted breast biopsy (VABB).

One of the first stereotactic devices was developed by Heywang-Koebrunner and Orel and colleagues in 1994 [16,33]. The Heywang-Koebrunner device allows MR imaging–guided breast biopsy in the prone or lateral decubitus position. The breast is compressed by two perforated plates with multiple horizontal holes that have MR-visible markers that serve as coordinates to calculate the lesion location. The coil allows horizontal access to the breast medially or laterally. Sterile bushings are used to protect the needle in the holes.

A similar stereotactic device has been developed by Kuhl and workers in cooperation with Philips Medical Systems [34]. This device is used with the patient in a semi-prone position. The perforated compression plates with a built-in stereotactic system immobilize the breast. The stereotactic system is integrated in a flexible circular surface coil, which is placed around the breast. A general disadvantage of stereotactic devices that use perforated compression plates is their limited pin-point accuracy. Lesions may be inaccessible if their path is hidden by a nonperforated area of the compression plates. The sterility of the compression plates is another problem.

A newly developed device overcomes most of these limitations (Fig. 2). This stereotactic device (MR-BI 160; Noras, Höchberg, Germany) can be integrated into a phased-array breast coil (open breast coil) (MRI-Devices/Invivo, Waukesha, Wisconsin) (Fig. 3). Alternatively and less costly, the system can be used with a special patient rest (MR-BI 160 PA; Noras, Höchberg, Germany) and a conventional ring or surface coil (Fig. 4). The procedure is performed with the patient in the prone position. The breast is compressed by a medial and lateral compression frame. These frames consist of flexible elastic bands that can be spread apart, avoiding any dead space. As an alternative, a grid positioning system is available. A guiding block with a needle carrier mounted on a guiding stick allows various needle angulations and access to all parts of the breast. A fluid-filled marker, which can be imaged, is used to calculate the coordinates of the lesion (Fig. 5). This apparatus and similar newly designed devices allow a more accurate needle placement and biopsy when compared with earlier devices.

Needles

Most MR imaging–guided biopsies are performed with the coaxial technique [50]. With this technique, a coaxial needle is placed under MR imaging

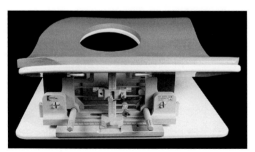

Fig. 3. The stereotactic system integrated into a phased-array breast coil which can be used for diagnostic imaging of the breast. (MRI Devices, Waukesha, WI.)

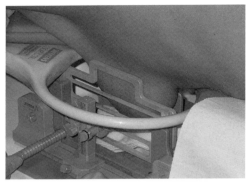

Fig. 4. The stereotactic system used together with a special patient rest (MR-BI 160PA Noras, Würzburg, Germany) and a ring coil (Siemens Medical Systems, Erlangen, Germany).

guidance, and biopsy is performed directly through it. Because the coaxial needle is used in the magnetic field of the unit, it must consist of nonmagnetic, MR imaging–compatible materials (eg, titanium).

As an alternative to the coaxial technique, the use of substitute needles has been described [49]. This needle type is placed under MR imaging guidance. After its correct position has been verified, it is replaced with the biopsy needle using the same coordinates on the aiming device. Because biopsy with coaxial techniques is easier to perform and more accurate, substitute needles are used less often.

After successful placement of the coaxial needle, biopsy needles are used to retrieve tissue specimens. A variety of biopsy needles of different shapes are available by several manufacturers (Table 2). Biopsy needles are not used in the magnetic field

(except with open magnets); therefore, they may consist of MR imaging–compatible as well as noncompatible materials (stainless steel [51]). Excellent results have been described using both materials (see Table 1); however, stainless steel needles are cheaper than dedicated MR imaging–compatible needles. In open magnets, the use of only fully MR imaging–compatible equipment is mandatory.

Techniques

Fine-needle aspiration biopsy

Fine-needle aspiration biopsy (FNAB) has been evaluated extensively using mammographic or sonographic guidance [52–54], and the limitations of this technique (eg, a high rate of insufficient samples) are well known. Reports on FNAB under MR guidance are limited [31,36,37,55]. Although satisfactory results were achieved in a study by Fischer and coworkers [36] who reported successful FNAB in 59 cases, most researchers suggest that FNAB has a low accuracy. Wald and coworkers [56] reported a 61% success rate in 18 patients with this technique only; therefore, FNAB under MR guidance, for which successful sampling must be guaranteed, cannot be recommended.

In contrast to FNAB, LCBB and VABB have been shown to be effective methods of diagnosing breast disorders and are reliable efficient alternatives to open surgical biopsy [18,20–22].

Large-core breast biopsy

Devices for MR imaging–guided LCBB are available from several manufacturers (Table 2) (Fig. 6). The patient is placed on the biopsy coil, and the breast is compressed in the mediolateral direction. In this position, a contrast-enhanced scan is performed.

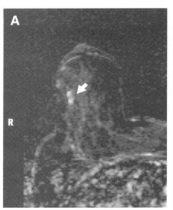 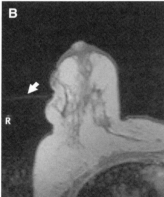 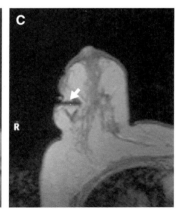

Fig. 5. (A) T1-weighted postcontrast images of a 64-year-old woman who presented with a suspicious enhancing lesion on MRI of the right breast. (B) Planning of the needle access to the focus. The fluid-filled marker (*arrow*) is used to calculate the coordinates of the lesion; it is shown as a hyperintense line. (see Fig. 1). (C) Control scan: coaxial needle approaches the lesion. Histology of the specimens revealed a fibroadenoma.

Table 2: **MRI-compatible devices for MR imaging-guided biopsy of breast lesions**

Manufacturer	Product	Technique
Somatex (Teltow, Germany)	Biopsy Handy	LCBB, 14–18G
Suros Surgical Systems (Indianapolis, Indiana)	ATEC	VABB, 9G, 12G
Invivo (Wuerzburg, Germany)	Double-Shoot Biopsy Gun	LCBB, 14–18G
	Semi-Automatic Biopsy Gun	LCBB, 14–18G
Bard (Murray Hill, New Jersey)	Vacora	VABB, 10G
Ethicon Endo-Surgery (Cincinatti, Ohio)	Mammotome MR	VABB, 9G, 12G, 14G

Based on these images, the coordinates of the lesion in the x, y, and z direction are calculated. These coordinates are transmitted on the aiming device of the biopsy unit. Usually, the angulation of the needle path is chosen in such a way that the needle is inserted parallel to the chest wall to avoid any injury to the chest wall and puncture of larger vessels. After local anesthesia, the coaxial needle is inserted and its correct position is checked in another unenhanced series. If necessary, the needle is repositioned until it approaches the target. When the optimal needle position is achieved, the patient is moved out of the magnet. Through the coaxial needle, a cutting LCBB needle is moved through the lesion. After each pass through the tissue, the needle is removed from the breast to obtain the specimen. A minimum of five specimens is recommended [57].

LCBB has been shown to yield good results (see Table 1); however, several potential limitations of this technique are known. First, retrieval of small lesions with LCBB can be difficult, possibly leading to incomplete characterization of the histologic findings. Second, MR imaging–guided breast biopsy has the problem of the "vanishing target." During the biopsy procedure, the lesion often becomes less conspicuous owing to washout of the contrast agent. For this reason, it would be helpful to acquire a larger volume of tissue in less time than is possible with 14-gauge LCBB needles. Third, LCBB needles do not readily provide a mechanism for placement of a localizing clip, which may be helpful for small lesions that undergo MR-guided biopsy.

Experiences with 14- to 16-gauge LCBB needles have been presented by several groups (Table 1) [34–36,51,58–60]. The largest series of MR imaging–guided LCBB has been presented by Kuhl and coworkers, who performed 14-gauge LCBB with a coaxial technique [35]. LCBB was technically successful in 77 of 78 (98%) of the lesions. One carcinoma was missed, and histologic underestimations were not observed. Similar results were presented by Chen and coworkers [51]. In 35 biopsies performed using 14-gauge LCBB, no missed carcinomas were reported, but two lesions were underestimated.

A new approach to LCBB has been developed by Pfleiderer and coworkers [61–63]. Their technique addresses the problem that the diagnosis of suspicious breast lesions and biopsy is always a two-step procedure. Diagnosis and simultaneous biopsy in a single examination would considerably reduce costs, save scanner time, and reduce strain on the patient, as well as reduce side effects. To achieve this goal, a robotic device has been developed by this group that is able to obtain a biopsy sample of breast lesions directly in the isocenter of a closed MR imaging scanner just after completion of the diagnostic study. To date, the second prototype of the device, called the ROBITOM (Robotic system for Biopsy and Interventional Therapy Of Mammary Lesions), has been presented. Experiments with tissue samples yielded a successful tissue harvest in 100%, and the group also reported successful LCBB in four patients [61]. Research is in progress to use this system, even in MR imaging–guided minimally invasive therapeutic interventions.

Vacuum-assisted breast biopsy

Similar to LCBB, most VABB procedures are performed with stereotactic systems using a coaxial technique. Three VABB systems are commercially available—the 10-gauge Vacora (Bard, Murray Hill, New Jersey) and the 9-gauge ATEC device (Suros Surgical Systems, Indianapolis, Indiana). An 11-gauge mammotome system (Ethicon Endo-surgery, Cincinnati, Ohio) has been used in several studies [64,65] (Table 2) (Figs. 7 and 8).

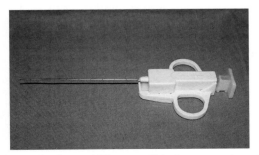

Fig. 6. Single-use MRI-compatible large-core breast biopsy device (Somatex, Teltow, Germany).

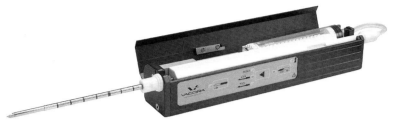

Fig. 7. MRI-compatible 10-gauge vacuum-assisted biopsy device (Bard Vacora, Bard Biopsy Systems, Tempe, AZ).

To target the lesion, a similar approach has been described as for LCBB. For the ATEC Vacora devices, coaxial needles and introducer sets are available by several manufacturers. The mammotome system has been used with coaxial needles as well as substitute needles.

VABB devices are attached to a vacuum that suctions tissue into a side window in the needle close to the needle tip. A rotating cutter advances over the tissue, cuts a core from the breast, and withdraws the specimen. By repeating these steps (tissue aspiration, cutting, and tissue retrieval) and by turning the needle clockwise around its axis, multiple cores are acquired. The vacuum always stays in place, and blood is suctioned out through the vacuum simultaneously (Figs. 9A–C, 10).

The advantages of VABB include a single probe insertion, directional sampling, and the ability to obtain more tissue in less time. These factors may be helpful, particularly in small lesions, and may provide better characterization of complex lesions (eg, lesions containing atypical ductal hyperplasia [ADH] and ductal carcinoma in situ [DCIS]). VABB also enables the placement of a localizing clip that can be used for subsequent needle localization under mammographic guidance.

Several studies have documented that VABB using a coaxial technique achieves a high diagnostic accuracy [32,64–67]. Extensive experience with MR-guided VABB has been presented by Perlet and colleagues. In a European multicenter study, 413 patients were referred for MR imaging–guided biopsies with an 11-gauge mammotome device [65]. In 72 of 413 lesions (17%), biopsy could not be performed for various reasons, including the fact that the lesion was no longer seen or had previously been incorrectly interpreted, or that problems occurred related to access or design of the biopsy coil. In 341 cases, biopsy was performed with an overall cancer yield of 25%. Seven lesions were initially missed at biopsy (2.0%); however, all of these cases could be immediately identified on post interventional images or because of radiologic-pathologic discordance. No late false-negative diagnoses occurred. Histologic underestimations were observed in three lesions. Complications were encountered in 16 of 341 lesions, including severe bleeding, infection, and vasovagal reaction.

Experience with a 9-gauge ATEC device was reported by Liberman in 2005 [68]. In 98 lesions on which biopsy was performed with this technique, four cancers were missed, and three lesions were underestimated. Nevertheless, all four false-negative lesions were retrospectively identified because of radiologic-pathologic discordance.

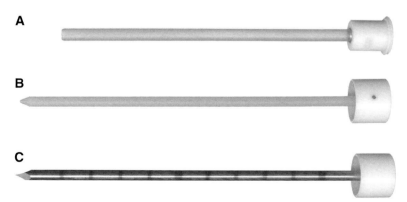

Fig. 8. MRI-compatible coaxial needle and introducer set for use with the Vacora Biopsy Device (Bard Biopsy Systems, Tempe, AZ).

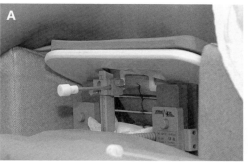
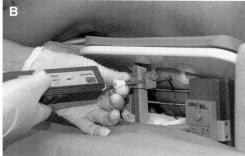
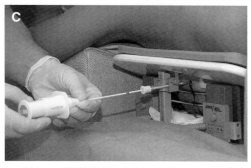

Fig. 9. (*A-C*): Vacuum-assisted breast biopsy (VABB). The intervention was performed with the stereotactic device described in **Fig. 1** and with the Vacora 10-gauge VABB system (BARD Biopsy Systems, Tempe, AZ). (*A*) Photograph shows the coaxial needle in situ. (*B*) Photograph shows the radiologist obtaining biopsy specimens. (*C*) Photograph shows clip placement through the coaxial needle.

Clip placement

At the completion of the biopsy, a clip marker should be placed through the coaxial sheath to mark the biopsy site so that the lesion can be localized in mammographic control studies or in the event that surgical removal of the area is necessary [69–71]. Complete removal of a lesion can occur in MR imaging–guided biopsy, and this is a more frequent event when larger tissue acquisition devices are used [72]. Nevertheless, complete removal of the imaging target does not ensure complete excision of the histologic process, and careful surgical and histologic evaluation of the biopsy site is necessary. MR-compatible clip markers are available

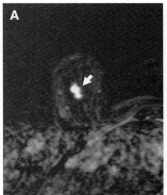
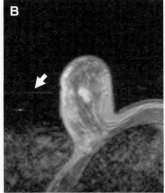
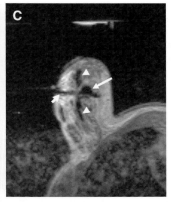

Fig. 10. (*A*) T1-weighted postcontrast images of a 55-year-old woman who presented with a suspicious enhancing lesion on MRI of the right breast. (*B*) Planning of the needle access to the focus. The fluid-filled marker (*arrow*) is used to calculate the coordinates of the lesion, it is shown as a hyperintense line. (see **Fig. 1**). (*C*) Post-interventional image shows the coaxial needle in situ (*small arrow*), bleeding within the tissue (*arrowheads*), and the biopsy cavity with the artefact of a metallic clip marker (*large arrow*). Histology of the specimens revealed infiltrating ductal carcinoma.

by several manufacturers (eg, MicroMark; Ethicon Endosurgery, Cincinnati, Ohio). A newly developed carbon-coated clip marker (BiomarC Tissue Marker; Carbon Medical Technologies, St. Paul, Minnesota) has been reported to have a low deployment rate [73]. In the study by Liberman and coworkers [66], clip placement (MammoMark Biopsy Site Marker; Artemis Medical, Heyward, California) following a VABB procedure was successful in 20 of 26 (77%) lesions at the initial attempt and was successful in another five lesions at a second attempt. The clip was evident as a low-signal focus with a median diameter of 0.6 cm on the MR images. In 19 of 25 lesions, the maximum distance from the clip to the biopsy site was 1 cm or less; in three lesions, this distance was 1.1 cm; and in three other lesions, the distance was greater than 3 cm.

MR imaging–guided breast biopsy in open magnets

Several groups have reported on MR imaging–guided LCBB in open magnets [39–41,43,74]. Two groups (Schneider and coworkers [39,40] and Sittek and coworkers [41]) used an open breast coil with a built-in biopsy device, that is, a special guidance device, whereas the third group used a free-hand method [43,44]. This free-hand approach was introduced by Daniel and colleagues in 2001. Because of the use of an open magnet, the biopsy needle can be visualized interactively during the insertion procedure, and interactive repositioning of the needle is possible until the needle tip is correctly placed at the edge of the target.

In all three groups, a high number of interventions were technically successful. In the studies by Schneider and Sittek, no cancer was missed, whereas with the free-hand method, one cancer was missed and two lesions were underestimated. All three studies evaluated a limited number of cases, and further investigation is necessary to assess definitively the potential advantages of biopsies in open magnets.

Comparison of the results

Research teams around the world have gained substantial experience with MR-guided biopsies. The data available in the literature document that MR-guided biopsy procedures can be performed successfully and accurately and should be offered as an adjunct to MR imaging of the breast. The best results have been described for techniques performed with stereotactic equipment using a coaxial technique. Excellent results have been obtained with LCBB and VABB. A high number of biopsies performed were technically successful (between 96.4% and 100.0%). The overall cancer yield of MR imaging–guided breast biopsy is reported to range from 23.5% to 47.5%. Reports of missed cancers vary widely, ranging from 0% to 16.6% (mean, 3.7%). False-negative rates are slightly higher for LCBB (5.5%) than for VABB (3.2%); however, the number of cases reported in the literature is limited, and, for a final assessment of the value of both techniques, further large-scale studies are needed. Because most lesions referred for MR imaging–guided biopsy are small, there may be an advantage for VABB, because this technique allows directional sampling and the retrieval of a greater tissue volume in less time. The frequency of histologic underestimation is reported to range from 0% to 25.0%, and the mean underestimation rates are 7.3% for LCBB and 5.3% for VABB. The reported results for MR imaging–guided breast biopsy are comparable to those obtained in breast biopsy under mammographic guidance, with reported false-negative rates of 0% to 8% for stereotactic 14-gauge LCBB and 1% to 3% for stereotactic 11-gauge VABB [18].

Patient management after MR imaging–guided breast biopsy

Despite careful interventional planning and a high standard of care, missed lesions at MR imaging–guided biopsy may occur. Radiologists should be aware of this fact, and several steps should be taken to prevent late false-negative results as much as possible.

Careful review of the images performed immediately after the biopsy is helpful to determine whether the lesion has been sampled. If these images suggest that the lesion has not been sampled, repositioning and additional tissue acquisition may be appropriate. If lesions exhibit rapid washout of the contrast material and review of the images after the procedure leaves doubt as to whether the lesion has been sampled, injection of a second dose of contrast material may be helpful. With this approach, complete removal of the MR imaging target was suggested in 57% and partial removal in 33% of 54 VABB procedures. In 10%, assessment was difficult owing to extensive bleeding [32]. In the European multicenter study published by Perlet and colleagues, seven lesions that were initially missed at biopsy could be identified on these post procedural images, and late false-negative results were completely avoided [65].

As a standard procedure after each MR imaging–guided biopsy, radiologists should retrospectively correlate the histologic results and imaging findings to ensure that the histology agrees with the morphology, signal behavior, and contrast enhancement of the lesion [75]. If needle biopsy yields a benign diagnosis concordant with the imaging findings, percutaneous biopsy can be considered accurate, and the patient is usually spared the need for open breast surgery. In these cases, a follow-up MR imaging study (usually after 6 months) is recommended [32]. In a study by Liberman and coworkers, four carcinomas that were initially missed at biopsy could be identified because of radiologic-pathologic discordance. Again, late false-negative results could be completely avoided [68].

Surgical excision is warranted for lesions that yield a percutaneous diagnosis of malignancy or a high-risk histology (eg, ADH or possible phyllodes tumor). Most groups report on underestimated cases in which ADH is diagnosed at percutaneous biopsy and DCIS is found at surgery, or DCIS is found at percutaneous biopsy and invasive cancer at surgery [51,65–67]. This phenomenon is well known from biopsy procedures performed under mammographic or sonographic guidance and underlines the importance of surgical excision of high-risk lesions.

In patients with discordant results, as well as in patients with uncertain assessment of the biopsy success, early follow-up MR imaging after 2 to 4 days (with the possibility of re-biopsy) or an open biopsy after MR imaging–guided wire localization is recommended [32].

Special attention should be paid to cases in which scheduled MR imaging–guided biopsy of a suspicious lesion is aborted owing to a lack of contrast enhancement at the date of the biopsy. Several groups have reported on such cases, and varying hormonal or inflammatory changes between the initial MR imaging and MR-guided biopsy most probably explain this phenomenon. In a study by Hefler and coworkers [76], 29 patients with no contrast enhancement at the date of the biopsy were followed up. In 4 of 29 patients, contrast enhancement reappeared within short-term follow-up, and three cases were found to be malignant.

Altogether, these data indicate that careful patient management after the biopsy is necessary. The data available in the literature indicate that a post procedural contrast-enhanced MR imaging study may be an appropriate tool to identify missed lesions. Together with radiologic-pathologic correlation, it should be possible to avoid many late false-negative diagnoses. In addition, the establishment of a quality assurance program for MR imaging–guided breast biopsy is useful to determine the level of care delivered by a facility and its individual physicians, to ensure that the equipment is functioning properly, and to help recognize problems as they arise so that they can be corrected.

From diagnosis to therapy: MR imaging–guided therapeutic interventions

With the early detection of small breast carcinomas, there has been an increasing interest in treatment with minimally invasive or even noninvasive imaging-guided methods [77–79]. To become generally accepted, these techniques must in the long term achieve equivalent or even better clinical outcomes than the traditional invasive methods. In the short term, these minimally invasive methods must show complete ablation of the lesion while leaving the surrounding normal tissue unaffected. The use of these techniques can also be justified by improving cosmesis and patient comfort and by reducing hospital stays and costs. Although some of these techniques have been described under mammographic and ultrasonographic guidance as well, MR imaging is the method of choice because it allows a more precise delineation of the lesion and assessment of the extent of the tumor.

Several techniques have been developed to achieve noninvasive or minimally invasive tumor ablation, including thermal ablation techniques, percutaneous excision under MR imaging guidance in open magnets, and interstitial radiotherapy. Thermal ablation techniques are based on the focused delivery of energy to the tumor tissue, which causes cell death, vascular obliteration, and tissue necrosis. Different approaches to thermal therapy have been described, including the use of ultrasonic waves (eg, focused ultrasound) and laser light (laser-light interstitial thermotherapy [LITT]). Some of these new approaches are discussed briefly herein.

Focused ultrasound is a completely noninvasive ablation method. Such waves have the potential to deliver energy precisely to a given point in soft tissue through the intact skin with an accuracy of 1 mm. Temperature elevations of 55° to 90°C at the focal spot are induced during a 10- to 20-second sonication. MR imaging can noninvasively measure the ultrasound-induced temperature because several MR parameters are temperature dependent. Initial in vivo studies in human breast cancer and fibroadenomas have shown promising results [80–84].

In LITT, MR imaging guidance is used to place thin optical fibers, which emit light from their tip, into the target region. These fibers are coupled to an Nd:YAG or semiconductor laser sources. LITT can be the direct extension of a breast biopsy because the fiber is commonly placed through the biopsy coaxial sheath. During LITT, a region of T1 hypointense signal appears around the optical fiber tip, which allows monitoring of the tissue necrosis. LITT has been used successfully for the treatment of benign fibroadenomas and is being studied as a treatment for breast cancer in several institutions [85–88].

The reverse effect is used in MR imaging–guided cryotherapy. Under MR imaging guidance, cryoprobes are inserted into the tumor bed with a target temperature of approximately −150°C. Similar to other techniques, cryotherapy leads to cellular death and vascular obliteration. Because of T2* shortening in frozen tissue, the expanding iceball appears as an increased area of signal void in MR images. Morin and coworkers [89] reported on 25 cryotherapies performed using a 0.5-T open magnet MR imager; 13 of 25 lesions were successfully treated.

When compared with percutaneous biopsy, minimally invasive therapeutic procedures are still in the preclinical stage of development. Although promising first results have been achieved, further research is necessary to expand the numerous pilot studies into large-scale clinical trials, with a study of long-term patient outcomes.

Summary

With the increasing use of diagnostic MR imaging of the breast, suspicious breast lesions that are occult at mammography and ultrasound can now be detected. For the histologic verification of such lesions, percutaneous MR imaging–guided biopsy techniques are available. The picture arising from the current literature is that MR imaging–guided percutaneous breast biopsy is safe and accurate, provided it is performed by an experienced physician with state-of-the-art equipment. Among the variety of systems and techniques, the best results have been described for stereotactic systems that allow precise interventions. Excellent results have been reported for LCBB and VABB; however, because lesions detected by MR imaging are often small, the authors see a certain advantage for VABB, which allows directional sampling and the retrieval of a greater tissue volume. A second important demand is accurate patient management after the intervention. Careful review of imaging and pathologic findings is strongly recommended. In addition, a post procedural contrast-enhanced MR imaging study seems helpful when uncertainty remains as to whether the lesion has been successfully sampled. Several newly developed devices and techniques, including interventions in open magnets and the use of robotic devices, require further investigation to assess their value.

Substantial effort has been made in the development of MR imaging–guided minimally invasive therapeutic procedures. Most of the studies that have evaluated these techniques have examined a limited number of cases, and long-term follow-up information is absent. Again, further investigation is required in this field.

References

[1] Bone B, Aspelin P, Bronge L, et al. Sensitivity and specificity of MR mammography with histopathological correlation in 250 breasts. Acta Radiol 1996;37:208–13.

[2] Fischer U, Kopka L, Grabbe E. Breast carcinoma: effect of preoperative contrast-enhanced MR imaging on the therapeutic approach. Radiology 1999;213:881–8.

[3] Gilles R, Guinebretiere JM, Lucidarme O, et al. Nonpalpable breast tumors: diagnosis with contrast-enhanced subtraction dynamic MR imaging. Radiology 1994;191:625–31.

[4] Helbich TH. Contrast-enhanced magnetic resonance imaging of the breast. Eur J Radiol 2000;34:208–19.

[5] Heywang SH, Wolf A, Pruss E, et al. MR imaging of the breast with Gd-DTPA: use and limitations. Radiology 1989;171:95–103.

[6] Heywang-Koebrunner SH, Viehweg P. Sensitivity of contrast-enhanced MR imaging of the breast. Magn Reson Imaging Clin N Am 1994;2:527–38.

[7] Kuhl CK. MRI of breast tumors. Eur Radiol 2000;10:46–58.

[8] Helbich TH, Becherer A, Trattnig S, et al. Differentiation of benign and malignant breast lesions: MR imaging versus Tc-99m sestamibi scintimammography. Radiology 1997;202:421–9.

[9] Ikeda DM. Progress report from the American College of Radiology Breast MR Imaging Lexicon Committee. Magn Reson Imaging Clin N Am 2001;9:295–302.

[10] Ikeda DM, Hylton NM, Kinkel K, et al. Development, standardization, and testing of a lexicon for reporting contrast-enhanced breast magnetic resonance imaging studies. J Magn Reson Imaging 2001;13:889–95.

[11] Kuhl CK, Mielcareck P, Klaschik S, et al. Dynamic breast MR imaging: are signal intensity time course data useful for differential diagnosis of enhancing lesions? Radiology 1999;211:101–10.

[12] Kuhl CK, Schild HH. Dynamic image interpretation of MRI of the breast. J Magn Reson Imaging 2000;12:965–74.

[13] Helbich TH, Roberts TP, Gossmann A, et al. Quantitative gadopentetate-enhanced MRI of breast tumors: testing of different analytic methods. Magn Reson Med 2000;44:915–24.

[14] Coulthard A. Magnetic resonance imaging-guided pre-operative breast localization using a "freehand technique." Br J Radiol 1996;69:482–3.

[15] Daniel BL, Birdwell RL, Ikeda DM, et al. Breast lesion localization: a freehand, interactive MR imaging-guided technique. Radiology 1998;207:455–63.

[16] Heywang-Kobrunner SH, Huynh AT, Viehweg P, et al. Prototype breast coil for MR-guided needle

localization. J Comput Assist Tomogr 1994;18: 876–81.

[17] Morris EA, Liberman L, Dershaw DD, et al. Preoperative MR imaging-guided needle localization of breast lesions. AJR Am J Roentgenol 2002; 178:1211–20.

[18] Helbich TH, Matzek W, Fuchsjager MH. Stereotactic and ultrasound-guided breast biopsy. Eur Radiol 2004;14:383–93.

[19] Parker SH, Burbank F, Jackman RJ, et al. Percutaneous large-core breast biopsy: a multi-institutional study. Radiology 1994;193:359–64.

[20] Liberman L. Centennial dissertation. Percutaneous imaging-guided core breast biopsy: state of the art at the millennium. AJR Am J Roentgenol 2000;174:1191–9.

[21] Pfarl G, Helbich TH, Riedl CC, et al. Stereotactic 11-gauge vacuum-assisted breast biopsy: a validation study. AJR Am J Roentgenol 2002;179: 1503–7.

[22] Memarsadeghi M, Pfarl G, Riedl C, et al. Value of 14-gauge ultrasound-guided large-core needle biopsy of breast lesions: own results in comparison with the literature. Rofo 2003;175:374–80.

[23] LaTrenta LR, Menell JH, Morris EA, et al. Breast lesions detected with MR imaging: utility and histopathologic importance of identification with US. Radiology 2003;227:856–61.

[24] Dhamanaskar KP, Muradall D. MRI directed ultrasound: a cost effective method for diagnosis and intervention in breast imaging [abstract]. Radiology 2002;225:653.

[25] Panizza P, De Gaspari A. Accuracy of post MR imaging second-look sonography in previously undetected breast lesions. [abstract]. Radiology 1997;205:489.

[26] Sickles EA, Parker SH. Appropriate role of core breast biopsy in the management of probably benign lesions. Radiology 1993;188:315.

[27] Graf O, Helbich TH, Fuchsjaeger MH, et al. Follow-up of palpable circumscribed noncalcified solid breast masses at mammography and US: can biopsy be averted? Radiology 2004;233: 850–6.

[28] Sickles EA. Probably benign breast lesions: when should follow-up be recommended and what is the optimal follow-up protocol? Radiology 1999; 213:11–4.

[29] Brenner RJ, Sickles EA. Surveillance mammography and stereotactic core breast biopsy for probably benign lesion: a cost comparison analysis. Acad Radiol 1997;4(6):419–25.

[30] Vizcaino I, Gadea L, Andreo L, et al. Short-term follow-up results in 795 nonpalpable probably benign lesions detected at screening mammography. Radiology 2001;219:475–83.

[31] Heywang-Kobrunner SH, Heinig A, Pickuth D, et al. Interventional MRI of the breast: lesion localisation and biopsy. Eur Radiol 2000;10:36–45.

[32] Heywang-Kobrunner SH, Heinig A, Schaumloffel U, et al. MR-guided percutaneous

excisional and incisional biopsy of breast lesions. Eur Radiol 1999;9:1656–65.

[33] Orel SG, Schnall MD, Newman RW, et al. MR imaging-guided localization and biopsy of breast lesions: initial experience. Radiology 1994;193: 97–102.

[34] Kuhl CK, Elevelt A, Leutner CC, et al. Interventional breast MR imaging: clinical use of a stereotactic localization and biopsy device. Radiology 1997;204:667–75.

[35] Kuhl CK, Morakkabati N, Leutner CC, et al. MR imaging–guided large-core (14-gauge) needle biopsy of small lesions visible at breast MR imaging alone. Radiology 2001;220:31–9.

[36] Fischer U, Kopka L, Grabbe E. Magnetic resonance guided localization and biopsy of suspicious breast lesions. Top Magn Reson Imaging 1998;9:44–59.

[37] Fischer U, Vosshenrich R, Doler W, et al. MR imaging-guided breast intervention: experience with two systems. Radiology 1995;195:533–8.

[38] Doler W, Fischer U, Metzger I, et al. Stereotaxic add-on device for MR-guided biopsy of breast lesions. Radiology 1996;200:863–4.

[39] Schneider JP, Schulz T, Horn LC, et al. MR-guided percutaneous core biopsy of small breast lesions: first experience with a vertically open 0.5 T scanner. J Magn Reson Imaging 2002;15: 374–85.

[40] Schneider JP, Schulz T, Ruger S, et al. MR-guided preoperative localization and percutaneous core biopsy of suspected breast lesions: possibilities and experience on the vertically open 0.5-T system. Radiologe 2002;42:33–41.

[41] Sittek H, Linsmeier E, Perlet C, et al. Preoperative marking and biopsy of nonpalpable breast lesions with a guidance system for the open Magnetom. Radiologe 2000;40:1098–105.

[42] Thiele J, Schneider JP, Franke P, et al. New method of MR-guided mammary biopsy. Rofo 1998;168:374–9.

[43] Daniel BL, Birdwell RL, Butts K, et al. Freehand iMRI-guided large-gauge core needle biopsy: a new minimally invasive technique for diagnosis of enhancing breast lesions. J Magn Reson Imaging 2001;13:896–902.

[44] Daniel BL, Freeman LJ, Pyzoha JM, et al. An MRI-compatible semiautomated vacuum-assisted breast biopsy system: initial feasibility study. J Magn Reson Imaging 2005;21:637–44.

[45] Kuhl CK, Bieling HB, Gieseke J, et al. Healthy premenopausal breast parenchyma in dynamic contrast-enhanced MR imaging of the breast: normal contrast medium enhancement and cyclical-phase dependency. Radiology 1997;203: 137–44.

[46] Muller-Schimpfle M, Ohmenhauser K, Stoll P, et al. Menstrual cycle and age: influence on parenchymal contrast medium enhancement in MR imaging of the breast. Radiology 1997;203: 145–9.

[47] Orel SG, Schnall MD. MR imaging of the breast for the detection, diagnosis, and staging of breast cancer. Radiology 2001;220:13–30.

[48] Helbich TH. Localization and biopsy of breast lesions by magnetic resonance imaging guidance. J Magn Reson Imaging 2001;13:903–11.

[49] Viehweg P, Heinig A, Amaya B, et al. MR-guided interventional breast procedures considering vacuum biopsy in particular. Eur J Radiol 2002; 42:32–9.

[50] Helbich TH, Mayr W, Schick S, et al. Coaxial technique: approach to breast core biopsies. Radiology 1997;203:684–90.

[51] Chen X, Lehman CD, Dee KE. MRI-guided breast biopsy: clinical experience with 14-gauge stainless steel core biopsy needle. AJR Am J Roentgenol 2004;182:1075–80.

[52] Howat AJ, Stringfellow HF, Briggs WA, et al. Fine needle aspiration cytology of the breast: a review of 1868 cases using the cytospin method. Acta Cytol 1994;38:939–44.

[53] Willis SL, Ramzy I. Analysis of false results in a series of 835 fine needle aspirates of breast lesions. Acta Cytol 1995;39:858–64.

[54] O'Neill SCM. Fine needle aspiration of 697 palpable breast lesions with histopathologic correlation. Surgery 1997;122:824–8.

[55] deSouza NM, Kormos DW, Krausz T, et al. MR-guided biopsy of the breast after lumpectomy and radiation therapy using two methods of immobilization in the lateral decubitus position. J Magn Reson Imaging 1995;5: 525–8.

[56] Wald DS, Weinreb JC, Newstead G, et al. MR-guided fine needle aspiration of breast lesions: initial experience. J Comput Assist Tomogr 1996;20:1–8.

[57] Liberman L. Stereotaxis 14-gauge breast biopsy: how many core biopsy specimens are needed? Radiology 1994;192:793–5.

[58] Veltman J, Boetes C, Wobbes T, et al. Magnetic resonance-guided biopsies and localizations of the breast: initial experiences using an open breast coil and compatible intervention device. Invest Radiol 2005;40:379–84.

[59] Lehman CD, Eby PR, Chen X, et al. MR imaging-guided breast biopsy using a coaxial technique with a 14-gauge stainless steel core biopsy needle and a titanium sheath. AJR Am J Roentgenol 2003;181:183–5.

[60] Fischer U, Rodenwaldt J, Hundertmark C, et al. MRI-assisted biopsy and localization of the breast. Radiologe 1997;37:692–701.

[61] Pfleiderer SO, Marx C, Vagner J, et al. Magnetic resonance-guided large-core breast biopsy inside a 1.5-T magnetic resonance scanner using an automatic system: in vitro experiments and preliminary clinical experience in four patients. Invest Radiol 2005;40:458–63.

[62] Pfleiderer SO, Reichenbach JR, Azhari T, et al. A manipulator system for 14-gauge large core breast biopsies inside a high-field whole-body MR scanner. J Magn Reson Imaging 2003;17: 493–8.

[63] Pfleiderer SO, Reichenbach JR, Wurdinger S, et al. Interventional MR-mammography: manipulator-assisted large core biopsy and interstitial laser therapy of tumors of the female breast. Z Med Phys 2003;13:198–202.

[64] Perlet C, Schneider P, Amaya B, et al. MR-guided vacuum biopsy of 206 contrast-enhancing breast lesions. Rofo 2002;174:88–95.

[65] Perlet C, Heinig A, Prat X, et al. Multicenter study for the evaluation of a dedicated biopsy device for MR-guided vacuum biopsy of the breast. Eur Radiol 2002;12:1463–70.

[66] Liberman L, Morris EA, Dershaw DD, et al. Fast MRI-guided vacuum-assisted breast biopsy: initial experience. AJR Am J Roentgenol 2003;181: 1283–93.

[67] Lehman CD, Deperi ER, Peacock S, et al. Clinical experience with MRI-guided vacuum-assisted breast biopsy. AJR Am J Roentgenol 2005;184: 1782–7.

[68] Liberman LBN. MRI-guided 9-gauge vacuum-assisted breast biopsy: initial clinical experience. AJR Am J Roentgenol 2005;185:183–93.

[69] Reynolds HE. Marker clip placement following directional, vacuum-assisted breast biopsy. Am Surg 1999;65:59–60.

[70] Burbank F, Forcier N. Tissue marking clip for stereotactic breast biopsy: initial placement accuracy, long-term stability, and usefulness as a guide for wire localization. Radiology 1997; 205:407–15.

[71] Liberman L, Dershaw DD, Morris EA, et al. Clip placement after stereotactic vacuum-assisted breast biopsy. Radiology 1997;205:417–22.

[72] Liberman L, Kaplan JB, Morris EA, et al. To excise or to sample the mammographic target: what is the goal of stereotactic 11-gauge vacuum-assisted breast biopsy? AJR Am J Roentgenol 2002;179: 679–83.

[73] Nelson MT, Garwood M, Meisamy S, et al. A new BiomarC tissue marker for breast biopsy: clinical evaluation in ultrasound, mammography, cat scanning and breast MR imaging [abstract]. Eur Radiol 2005;15:298.

[74] Sittek H, Perlet C, Herrmann K, et al. MR mammography: preoperative marking of non-palpable breast lesions with the Magnetom open at 0.2 T. Radiologe 1997;37:685–91.

[75] Liberman L. Clinical management issues in percutaneous core breast biopsy. Radiol Clin North Am 2000;38:791–807.

[76] Hefler L, Casselman J, Amaya B, et al. Follow-up of breast lesions detected by MRI not biopsied due to absent enhancement of contrast medium. Eur Radiol 2003;13:344–6.

[77] Kacher DF, Jolesz FA. MR imaging–guided breast ablative therapy. Radiol Clin North Am 2004;42: 947–62.

[78] Hall-Craggs MA. Interventional MRI of the breast: minimally invasive therapy. Eur Radiol 2000;10:59–62.

[79] Singletary SE. Minimally invasive ablation techniques in breast cancer treatment. Ann Surg Oncol 2002;9:319–20.

[80] Zippel DB, Papa MZ. The use of MR imaging guided focused ultrasound in breast cancer patients: a preliminary phase one study and review. Breast Cancer 2005;12:32–8.

[81] Huber PE, Jenne JW, Rastert R, et al. A new noninvasive approach in breast cancer therapy using magnetic resonance imaging-guided focused ultrasound surgery. Cancer Res 2001;61: 8441–7.

[82] Hynynen K, Pomeroy O, Smith DN, et al. MR imaging-guided focused ultrasound surgery of fibroadenomas in the breast: a feasibility study. Radiology 2001;219:176–85.

[83] Gianfelice D, Khiat A, Amara M, et al. MR imaging-guided focused ultrasound surgery of breast cancer: correlation of dynamic contrast-enhanced MRI with histopathologic findings. Breast Cancer Res Treat 2003;82:93–101.

[84] Gianfelice D, Khiat A, Amara M, et al. MR imaging-guided focused US ablation of breast cancer: histopathologic assessment of effectiveness—initial experience. Radiology 2003;227:849–55.

[85] Harms SMH. MRI directed interstitial thermal ablation of breast fibroadenomas. [abstract 362]. In: Seventh Proceedings of the International Society of Magnetic Resonance Medicine. Hoboken (NJ): Wiley & Sons; 1999.

[86] Mumtaz H, Hall-Craggs MA, Wotherspoon A, et al. Laser therapy for breast cancer: MR imaging and histopathologic correlation. Radiology 1996;200:651–8.

[87] Dowlatshahi K, Francescatti DS, Bloom KJ. Laser therapy for small breast cancers. Am J Surg 2002; 184:359–63.

[88] Dowlatshahi K, Fan M, Gould VE, et al. Stereotactically guided laser therapy of occult breast tumors: work-in-progress report. Arch Surg 2000; 135:1345–52.

[89] Morin J, Traore A, Dionne G, et al. Magnetic resonance-guided percutaneous cryosurgery of breast carcinoma: technique and early clinical results. Can J Surg 2004;47:347–51.

ELSEVIER
SAUNDERS

MAGNETIC
RESONANCE
IMAGING CLINICS

Magn Reson Imaging Clin N Am 14 (2006) 427–430

Index

Note: Page numbers of article titles are in **boldface** type.

Moving?

Make sure your subscription moves with you!

To notify us of your new address, find your **Clinics Account Number** (located on your mailing label above your name), and contact customer service at:

E-mail: elspcs@elsevier.com

800-654-2452 (subscribers in the U.S. & Canada)
407-345-4000 (subscribers outside of the U.S. & Canada)

Fax number: 407-363-9661

Elsevier Periodicals Customer Service
6277 Sea Harbor Drive
Orlando, FL 32887-4800

*To ensure uninterrupted delivery of your subscription, please notify us at least 4 weeks in advance of move.